The Ultimate Renal Diet Cookbook for Seniors

110 KIDNEY-FRIENDLY RECIPES, 60-DAY MEAL PLAN, AND
COMPREHENSIVE SHOPPING LIST FOR A HEALTHY LIFESTYLE

ABIGAIL BUTLER

TABLE OF CONTENTS

TABLE OF CONTENTS

INTRODUCTION TO THE RENAL DIET

When navigating kidney health, understanding how diet impacts your well-being is essential. A renal diet is specifically designed to reduce the workload on your kidneys, helping to maintain their function and prevent further complications. The significance of a renal diet, its objectives, and how it may be easily included in your senior lifestyle will all be covered in this introduction.

Why Is the Renal Diet Important?

Your kidneys are essential for removing waste and extra fluid from your circulation. Waste can accumulate in your body when kidney function is impaired, which can result in a number of health issues. By limiting the consumption of specific minerals that might put stress on the kidneys, such as salt, potassium, and phosphorus, a renal diet helps manage these problems. A well-planned renal diet can:

- **Reduce the strain on your kidneys to support renal function.**
- **Control symptoms** such as swelling, high blood pressure, or fatigue.
- **Prevent complications** like bone disease or heart problems.
- **Improve overall quality of life,** making every day more manageable and enjoyable.

Who Benefits from a Renal Diet?

For those with chronic kidney disease (CKD), especially in its early stages, this diet is most helpful.
Seniors, in particular, can gain immense value from this approach, as aging can naturally affect kidney function. Even if you're not yet experiencing significant symptoms, adopting a renal-friendly diet early can help slow disease progression and maintain your independence.

Core Principles of the Renal Diet

The renal diet focuses on moderation and balance. Key principles include:

- **Controlling Sodium:** Helps manage blood pressure and reduces swelling.
- **Regulating Potassium:** Maintains a healthy heart rhythm and prevents dangerous levels from building up in your blood.
- **Managing Phosphorus:** Protects bone health and reduces risks associated with high phosphorus levels.
- **Moderating Protein Intake:** Reduces the production of waste that the kidneys must filter while still providing essential nutrients for muscle maintenance.

By prioritizing these principles, the renal diet becomes a powerful tool in managing kidney health while allowing room for creativity and enjoyment in your meals.

NUTRITIONAL GUIDELINES FOR SENIORS

Seniors have unique nutritional needs, especially when managing kidney health. This chapter focuses on the dietary adjustments required for optimal kidney function, alongside considerations for age-related nutritional requirements.

Understanding Nutritional Challenges for Seniors

Age-related changes in our bodies can have an impact on nutrition, including:

- **Reduced Appetite:** Due to slower metabolism or medical conditions.
- **Difficulty Chewing or Swallowing:** Making some foods less accessible.
- **Altered Taste Sensation:** This can affect food preferences.
- **Nutrient Absorption Issues:** Particularly for vitamins like B12 and calcium.

When managing kidney health, these factors must be considered alongside the restrictions of a renal diet to ensure you receive adequate nutrition.

Key Nutrients to Monitor

Sodium

- **Why It Matters:** Excess sodium can lead to fluid retention, high blood pressure, and added stress on your kidneys.
- **Guidelines:** Limit sodium intake to less than 2,000 mg per day.
- **Tips:** Use herbs, spices, and low-sodium alternatives to enhance flavor.

Potassium

- **Why It Matters:** High potassium levels can cause heart irregularities and muscle weakness.
- **Guidelines:** Keep potassium intake within recommended limits (discuss with your healthcare provider).
- **Tips:** Opt for low-potassium fruits and vegetables like apples, berries, and green beans.

Phosphorus

- **Why It Matters:** High phosphorus levels can lead to weakened bones and calcium deposits in tissues.
- **Guidelines:** Restrict phosphorus intake by avoiding processed foods and choosing fresh options.
- **Tips:** Look for phosphate additives on labels and avoid foods like dark sodas and processed cheeses.

Protein

- **Why It Matters:** While protein is essent ial, too much can increase waste products in your blood.
- **Guidelines:** Aim for high-quality protein sources in moderation, like lean meats, eggs, and tofu.
- **Tips:** Balance protein intake with other nutrient-rich foods.

Fluid Intake

- **Why It Matters:** Excess fluid can build up, causing swelling and added strain on the heart.
- **Guidelines:** Monitor fluid intake as directed by your healthcare provider.
- **Tips:** Use small cups and track your daily fluid consumption.

Balancing Nutrition and Enjoyment

While restrictions may feel overwhelming, they don't mean sacrificing enjoyment at mealtimes. By focusing on fresh, natural ingredients and experimenting with flavors, you can create meals that are both kidney-friendly and satisfying.

HOW TO USE THIS COOKBOOK

This cookbook is designed to simplify your journey toward better kidney health. With user-friendly recipes, meal plans, and practical tips, you'll find everything you need to make kidney-friendly eating effortless and enjoyable.

Getting Started

Before diving into the recipes, take time to familiarize yourself with the key features of this cookbook:

- **Recipe Sections:** Organized by meal type, including breakfasts, lunches, dinners, snacks, and desserts.
- **Nutritional Information:** Each recipe includes detailed data on sodium, potassium, phosphorus, protein, and calories.
- **Dietary Tips:** Look for highlighted tips to make recipes even more suitable for your dietary needs.

The 60-Day Meal Plan

One of the standout features of this cookbook is the 60-day meal plan, which:

- Provides structure to your daily meals.
- Ensures balanced nutrition.
- Eliminates the stress of meal planning.

Start with the **First-Week Shopping List** to stock your kitchen with essentials. This detailed list includes everything you need for your first week of meals, ensuring a smooth transition into kidney-friendly eating.

Adapting Recipes to Your Needs

While all recipes are tailored to be renal-friendly, individual needs may vary. Use these tips to adapt recipes:

- **Adjust Portion Sizes** based on your daily caloric and nutrient requirements.
- **Swap Ingredients:** For example, substitute higher-potassium vegetables with lower-potassium alternatives.
- **Consult Your Dietitian:** When in doubt, discuss modifications with a healthcare professional.

Cooking Tips for Seniors

To make cooking more manageable:

- **Simplify Prep:** Choose recipes with minimal chopping or complex techniques.
- **Batch Cook:** Prepare larger portions to save time during the week.
- **Use Assistive Tools,** such as ergonomic utensils or food processors.

Enjoying the Process

Remember, this journey is about rediscovering the joy of eating while caring for your health. Experiment with new flavors, involve loved ones in the cooking process and celebrate small victories along the way.

With this cookbook, you have a comprehensive guide to making kidney-friendly living not only manageable but truly enjoyable. Let's take the first step together toward a healthier, happier you!

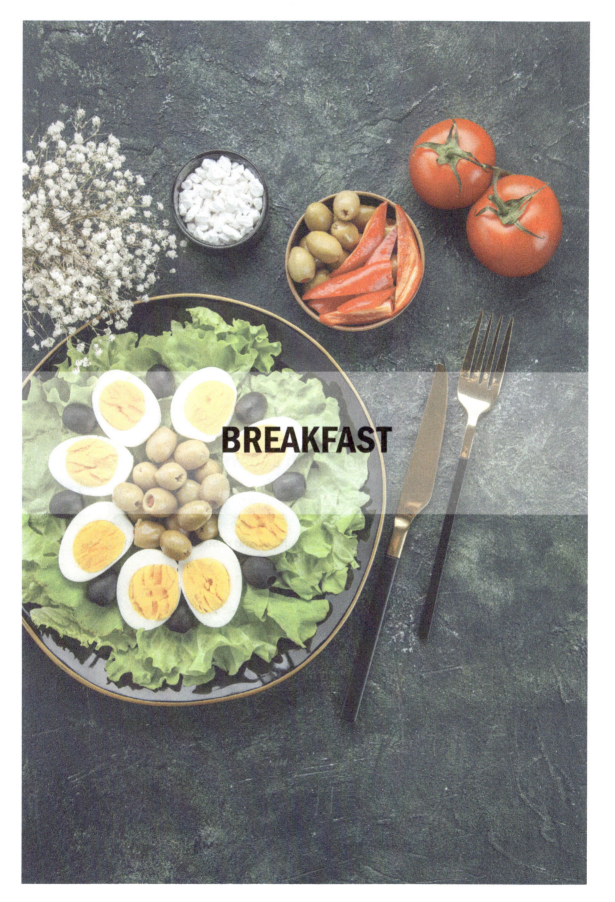

BREAKFAST

QUINOA BREAKFAST BOWL WITH FRUIT

 **PREP TIME:** 5 minutes   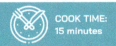 **COOK TIME:** 15 minutes   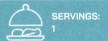 **SERVINGS:** 1

A wholesome and nourishing breakfast bowl with protein-rich quinoa and fresh fruits.

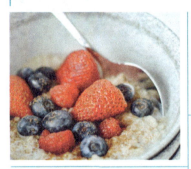

INGREDIENTS:

- 1/4 cup uncooked quinoa (43 g)
- 1/2 cup water (120 mL)
- One-fourth cup (60 mL) of unsweetened almond milk
- 1/4 cup fresh blueberries (40 g)
- 1/4 cup diced strawberries (40 g)
- 1/4 teaspoon cinnamon (0.5 g)

INSTRUCTIONS:

1. To get rid of any bitterness, rinse the quinoa with cold water.
2. Rinse the quinoa and add the water to a small saucepan. Bring to a boil over medium heat.
3. For 12 to 15 minutes or when the quinoa is soft and the water has been absorbed, lower the heat to low, cover, and simmer.
4. Stir in the almond milk and cinnamon. Cook over low heat until creamy, about 2 more minutes.
5. After taking the quinoa off of the stove, pour it into a serving bowl.
6. Top the quinoa with the fresh blueberries and diced strawberries.
7. Serve warm, and enjoy immediately.

NUTRITIONAL:
Calories: 180
Protein: 5 g
Fat: 3 g
Carbohydrates: 30 g
Sodium: 10 mg
Potassium: 120 mg
Phosphorus: 60 mg

CUCUMBER AND EGG WRAP

 **PREP TIME:** 5 minutes   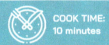 **COOK TIME:** 10 minutes   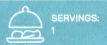 **SERVINGS:** 1

A simple and nutritious wrap combining fresh cucumber and protein-packed egg whites.

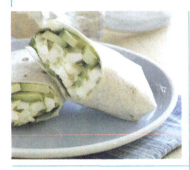

INGREDIENTS:

- 1 low-sodium tortilla (30 g)
- 2 boiled egg whites, sliced (1/4 cup / 60 g)
- 1/4 cup peeled and thinly sliced cucumber (30 g)
- 1/8 teaspoon ground black pepper (0.3 g)

INSTRUCTIONS:

1. Lay the low-sodium tortilla flat on a clean surface.
2. Arrange the sliced boiled egg whites evenly in the center of the tortilla.
3. Add the peeled and thinly sliced cucumber on top of the egg whites.
4. Sprinkle the black pepper evenly over the filling.
5. Make sure the filling is secure by rolling the tortilla tightly around it.
6. Slice the wrap in half, if desired, and serve immediately.

NUTRITIONAL:
Calories: 80
Protein: 6 g
Fat: 1 g
Carbohydrates: 10 g
Sodium: 35 mg
Potassium: 50 mg
Phosphorus: 25 mg

TOFU SCRAMBLE

 **PREP TIME:** 5 minutes   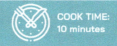 **COOK TIME:** 10 minutes   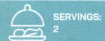 **SERVINGS:** 2

A hearty and flavorful plant-based scramble made with tofu and colorful red bell pepper.

INGREDIENTS:

- 1/2 block firm tofu (low potassium, about 150 g)
- 1/4 teaspoon turmeric powder (0.5 g)
- 1/4 cup diced red bell pepper (40 g)
- 1 teaspoon olive oil (5 mL)

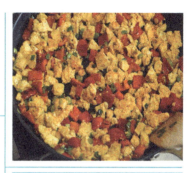

INSTRUCTIONS:

1. After draining, use a fresh towel to pat the tofu dry. Rumble it with a fork or your hands into tiny, bite-sized pieces.
2. Reheat the olive oil in a non-stick skillet over medium heat.
3. Put the diced red bell pepper in the skillet and sauté for 2 to 3 minutes or until slightly softened.
4. Put the crumbled tofu in the skillet and sprinkle the turmeric powder over it. Stir well to combine.
5. The tofu should be cooked through and gently browned after 5 to 7 minutes of cooking, stirring periodically.
6. Replace the heat and transfer the tofu scramble to serving plates.
7. Serve warm, optionally garnished with fresh herbs like parsley or chives.

Calories: 80
Protein: 7 g
Fat: 4 g
Carbohydrates: 3 g
Sodium: 10 mg
Potassium: 60 mg
Phosphorus: 40 mg

NUTRITIONAL:

VEGGIE OMELETTE

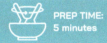 **PREP TIME:** 5 minutes   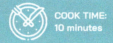 **COOK TIME:** 10 minutes   **SERVINGS:** 1

A light and flavorful omelette packed with kidney-friendly vegetables.

INGREDIENTS:

- 4 egg whites or two large eggs (4 oz / 120 g total)
- 1/4 cup diced red bell pepper (40 g)
- 2 tablespoons finely chopped onion (20 g)
- 1 teaspoon olive oil (5 mL)
- 1/8 teaspoon ground black pepper (0.3 g)

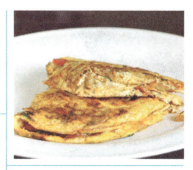

INSTRUCTIONS:

1. In a small-sized bowl, crack the eggs and whisk until smooth. Mix well after adding the black pepper.
2. Reheat the olive oil in a non-stick skillet over medium heat. Swirl the pan to distribute the oil on the bottom.
3. Add the red bell pepper and chopped onion to the pan. Sauté for 2 to 3 minutes until the vegetables soften.
4. Pour the whisked eggs or egg whites over the vegetables in the skillet. Let the mixture cook undisturbed for about 2 minutes or until the edges start to set.
5. To let the raw egg run below, carefully raise one edge of the omelette with a spatula. Cook until the eggs are set, about 2 more minutes.
6. Slide the omelette onto a plate after carefully folding it in half. Warm up and serve.

Calories: 140
Protein: 12 g
Fat: 9 g
Carbohydrates: 4 g
Sodium: 75 mg
Potassium: 150 mg
Phosphorus: 125 mg

NUTRITIONAL:

GREEN SHAKSHUKA

PREP TIME:
10 minutes

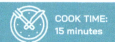
COOK TIME:
15 minutes

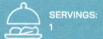
SERVINGS:
1

An herby twist on a classic dish, this kidney-friendly green shakshuka is both nourishing and delicious.

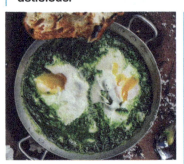

INGREDIENTS:

- 2 large eggs or 4 egg whites (4 oz / 120 g total)
- 1/2 cup chopped spinach (20 g)
- 1/4 cup chopped zucchini (40 g)
- 2 tablespoons finely chopped green onion (20 g)
- 1 teaspoon olive oil (5 mL)
- 1/8 teaspoon ground black pepper (0.3 g)
- 1/4 teaspoon ground cumin (optional, 0.5 g)

INSTRUCTIONS:

1. In a small bowl, crack the eggs and whisk until smooth. Add the ground black pepper and cumin, if using, and mix well.
2. Heat the olive oil in a non-stick skillet over medium heat. Swirl the pan to coat the bottom.
3. Add the chopped zucchini and green onion to the skillet. Sauté for 2 to 3 minutes until softened.
4. Stir in the spinach and cook for an additional 1 to 2 minutes until wilted.
5. Pour the whisked eggs or egg whites evenly over the vegetables. Allow the mixture to cook undisturbed for about 2 minutes or until the edges begin to set.
6. Using a spatula, gently lift the edges of the mixture to allow the raw egg to flow underneath. Cook until the eggs are set, about 2 to 3 more minutes.
7. Slide the shakshuka onto a plate or serve directly from the skillet. Enjoy warm.

NUTRITIONAL:
Calories: 135
Protein: 12 g
Fat: 8 g
Carbohydrates: 3 g
Sodium: 80 mg
Potassium: 130 mg
Phosphorus: 120 mg

BLUEBERRY OATMEAL

PREP TIME:
5 minutes

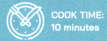
COOK TIME:
10 minutes

SERVINGS:
1

A warm, cozy breakfast dish with a touch of cinnamon and the sweetness of fresh blueberries.

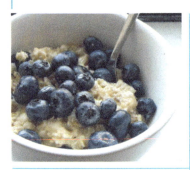

INGREDIENTS:

- 1/2 cup rolled oats (40 g)
- 1 cup unsweetened almond milk (240 mL)
- 1/4 cup fresh blueberries (40 g)
- 1/4 teaspoon ground cinnamon (0.5 g)

INSTRUCTIONS:

1. Mix the rolled oats and almond milk in a small saucepan. Stir to mix evenly.
2. Put the saucepan over medium heat and bring the contents to a moderate boil. Stir occasionally to prevent sticking.
3. Turn the heat down to low and simmer the oatmeal for 5 to 7 minutes or until the oats are soft and the consistency you want is achieved.
4. Replace the saucepan from the heat and stir in the ground cinnamon. Mix well.
5. Replace the oatmeal in a serving bowl and top with the fresh blueberries.
6. Serve warm, and enjoy immediately.

NUTRITIONAL:
Calories: 150
Protein: 4 g
Fat: 3 g
Carbohydrates: 26 g
Sodium: 75 mg
Potassium: 120 mg
Phosphorus: 100 mg

APPLE CINNAMON SMOOTHIE

 **PREP TIME:** 5 minutes   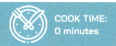 **COOK TIME:** 0 minutes   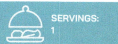 **SERVINGS:** 1

A creamy and refreshing smoothie with the comforting flavors of apple and cinnamon.

INGREDIENTS:

- 1 cup unsweetened almond milk (240 mL)
- 1 medium peeled apple, chopped (about 150 g)
- 1/4 teaspoon ground cinnamon (0.5 g)
- 1/2 cup ice cubes (120 mL)

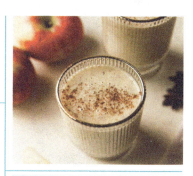

INSTRUCTIONS:

1. Cut the apple into little pieces after peeling it.
2. Add the unsweetened almond milk, chopped apple, ground cinnamon, and ice cubes to a blender.
3. For one to two minutes or until the mixture is creamy and smooth, blend on high speed.
4. Pour the smoothie into a glass.
5. Serve immediately and enjoy.

Calories: 80
Protein: 1 g
Fat: 2 g
Carbohydrates: 15 g
Sodium: 70 mg
Potassium: 120 mg
Phosphorus: 20 mg

NUTRITIONAL:

AVOCADO TOAST

 **PREP TIME:** 5 minutes   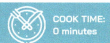 **COOK TIME:** 0 minutes   **SERVINGS:** 1

A simple and satisfying toast with creamy avocado, a hint of lemon, and black pepper.

INGREDIENTS:

- 1 slice low-sodium bread (30 g)
- 1 to 2 thin slices of avocado (20 g)
- 1/2 teaspoon lemon juice (2.5 mL)
- 1/8 teaspoon ground black pepper (0.3 g)

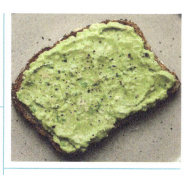

INSTRUCTIONS:

1. Toast the low-sodium bread to your desired level of crispness.
2. Using a fork, carefully distribute the avocado slices on top of the toast.
3. Drizzle the lemon juice evenly over the avocado.
4. Sprinkle the black pepper on top to season.
5. Serve immediately and enjoy.

Calories: 90
Protein: 2 g
Fat: 5 g
Carbohydrates: 10 g
Sodium: 30 mg
Potassium: 120 mg
Phosphorus: 30 mg

NUTRITIONAL:

RICE PORRIDGE WITH BANANA

 **PREP TIME:** 5 minutes   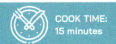 **COOK TIME:** 15 minutes   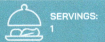 **SERVINGS:** 1

A warm and creamy porridge made with white rice and a touch of natural sweetness from banana.

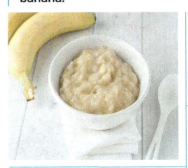

INGREDIENTS:

- 1/4 cup uncooked white rice (50 g)
- 1 cup water (240 mL)
- One-fourth cup (60 mL) of unsweetened almond milk
- 2 tablespoons mashed banana (30 g)

INSTRUCTIONS:

1. Rinse the white rice under cold water to remove excess starch.
2. Put the rice and water in a small pot. Over medium heat, bring the mixture to a boil.
3. Lid the pot, lower the heat to low, and simmer the rice for 12 to 15 minutes or until it is tender and most of the water has been absorbed.
4. Stir in the almond milk and continue cooking for 2 minutes, stirring occasionally, until the porridge reaches a creamy consistency.
5. Replace the saucepan from the heat and gently fold in the mashed banana. Mix well to combine.
6. Replace the porridge with a serving bowl and let it cool slightly before serving.

NUTRITIONAL:
Calories: 120
Protein: 2 g
Fat: 1 g
Carbohydrates: 25 g
Sodium: 5 mg
Potassium: 80 mg
Phosphorus: 30 mg

ZUCCHINI PANCAKES

 **PREP TIME:** 10 minutes    **COOK TIME:** 10 minutes   **SERVINGS:** 2

Light and savory pancakes made with fresh zucchini and a touch of olive oil.

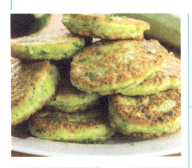

INGREDIENTS:

- 1 cup grated zucchini (150 g)
- Two egg whites (60 mL or 1/4 cup)
- 1/4 cup all-purpose flour (30 g)
- 1 tablespoon olive oil (15 mL)

INSTRUCTIONS:

1. Place the zucchini on a fresh kitchen towel after grating it using a box grater. Move the zucchini to a mixing dish after squeezing out any extra liquid.
2. Add the egg whites and all-purpose flour to the bowl with the zucchini. Stir until the ingredients are well combined.
3. Heat half of the olive oil in a non-stick skillet over medium heat.
4. For each pancake, use the back of a spoon to gently press about 2 teaspoons of the zucchini mixture into the skillet.
5. Cook until it becomes golden brown on one side for 3 minutes; flip and cook for another 2 to 3 minutes.
6. Continue with the leftover zucchini mixture, adjusting the amount of olive oil as necessary.
7. Replace the pancakes on a plate and serve warm.

NUTRITIONAL:
Calories: 110
Protein: 4 g
Fat: 6 g
Carbohydrates: 10 g
Sodium: 5 mg
Potassium: 150 mg
Phosphorus: 35 mg

CHIA BERRY PUDDING

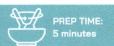 **PREP TIME:** 5 minutes

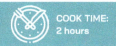 **COOK TIME:** 2 hours

 SERVINGS: 1

A creamy and refreshing pudding made with chia seeds and the natural sweetness of strawberries.

INGREDIENTS:

- 1 tablespoon chia seeds (10 g)
- 1/2 cup of unsweetened almond milk (120 mL)
- 2 strawberries, chopped (30 g)
- 1/4 teaspoon vanilla extract (1.25 mL)

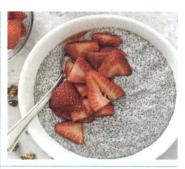

INSTRUCTIONS:

1. In a small-sized bowl, mix the chia seeds, almond milk, and vanilla extract. Stir well to ensure the chia seeds are evenly distributed.
2. Top the bowl or jar and place it in the refrigerator for at least 2 hours or until the mixture thickens into a pudding-like consistency.
3. Once the pudding is set, stir it again to break up any clumps.
4. Top the chia pudding with the sliced strawberries.
5. Serve right now or store in the refrigerator until you're ready to eat.

NUTRITIONAL:
Calories: 80
Protein: 2 g
Fat: 3 g
Carbohydrates: 8 g
Sodium: 30 mg
Potassium: 80 mg
Phosphorus: 50 mg

BREAKFAST RICE BOWL

 **PREP TIME:** 5 minutes

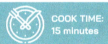 **COOK TIME:** 15 minutes

 SERVINGS: 1

A simple and satisfying breakfast bowl featuring fluffy white rice and sautéed red bell pepper.

INGREDIENTS:

- 1/2 cup cooked white rice (85 g)
- 1/4 cup diced red bell pepper (40 g)
- 1 teaspoon olive oil (5 mL)
- 1/8 teaspoon ground black pepper (0.3 g)

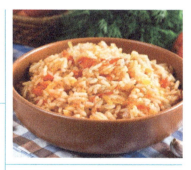

INSTRUCTIONS:

1. If you haven't already, cook the white rice as directed on the package.
2. Reheat the olive oil in a small, non-stick skillet over medium heat.
3. Put the chopped red bell pepper in the pan and cook until it softens slightly, about 3 minutes.
4. Put the cooked white rice in the pan with the peppers. Stir gently to mix and cook the rice thoroughly.
5. Sprinkle the black pepper over the mixture and stir again.
6. Transfer the rice and pepper mixture to a serving bowl. Serve warm.

NUTRITIONAL:
Calories: 130
Protein: 2 g
Fat: 2 g
Carbohydrates: 26 g
Sodium: 5 mg
Potassium: 50 mg
Phosphorus: 20 mg

CINNAMON FRENCH TOAST

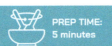 **PREP TIME:** 5 minutes   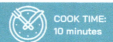 **COOK TIME:** 10 minutes   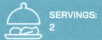 **SERVINGS:** 2

A classic breakfast favorite made kidney-friendly with low-sodium bread and a touch of cinnamon.

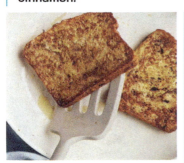

INGREDIENTS:

- 2 slices low-sodium bread (60 g)
- 2 egg whites (1/4 cup or 60 mL)
- 1/4 cup of unsweetened almond milk (60 mL)
- 1/4 teaspoon ground cinnamon (0.5 g)

INSTRUCTIONS:

1. Beat the egg whites, almond milk, and ground cinnamon together in a shallow bowl until thoroughly blended.
2. Preheat a non-stick skillet over medium heat. If needed, lightly coat with a small amount of olive oil or cooking spray.
3. Make sure both sides of one piece of bread are equally coated after dipping it into the egg mixture.
4. Place the coated bread onto the skillet and cook for 2 to 3 minutes on one side or until golden brown.
5. Cook for a further two to three minutes after flipping the bread or until the opposite side is golden brown.
6. Repeat the process with the second slice of bread.
7. Before serving, move the French toast to a platter and allow it to cool somewhat.

NUTRITIONAL:
Calories: 90
Protein: 5 g
Fat: 2 g
Carbohydrates: 12 g
Sodium: 40 mg
Potassium: 60 mg
Phosphorus: 25 mg

SMOOTHIE BOWL

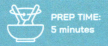 **PREP TIME:** 5 minutes   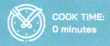 **COOK TIME:** 0 minutes   **SERVINGS:** 1

A refreshing and creamy smoothie bowl with tropical pineapple and vibrant raspberries.

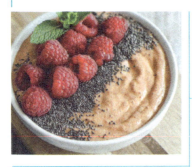

INGREDIENTS:

- 1/2 cup frozen pineapple chunks (75 g)
- 1/4 cup coconut milk (60 mL)
- 1/4 cup fresh raspberries (30 g)
- 1 teaspoon chia seeds (optional, 5 g)

INSTRUCTIONS:

1. Place the frozen pineapple chunks and coconut milk in a blender. Blend until smooth and creamy.
2. Using a spoon, evenly distribute the smoothie mixture after pouring it into a bowl.
3. Top the smoothie base with the fresh raspberries and sprinkle the chia seeds on top, if using.
4. Serve immediately with a spoon, and enjoy.

NUTRITIONAL:
Calories: 110
Protein: 1 g
Fat: 5 g
Carbohydrates: 15 g
Sodium: 10 mg
Potassium: 80 mg
Phosphorus: 20 mg

EGG AND BELL PEPPER MUFFINS

 **PREP TIME:** 10 minutes 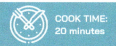 **COOK TIME:** 20 minutes 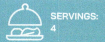 **SERVINGS:** 4

Light and protein-packed muffins with the vibrant flavor of red bell pepper.

INGREDIENTS:

- 4 large egg whites (1/2 cup / 120 mL)
- 1/2 cup red bell pepper, diced (75 g)
- 1 teaspoon olive oil (5 mL)

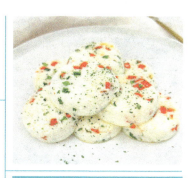

INSTRUCTIONS:

1. Reheat the oven to 350°F (or 175°C). Use silicone muffin liners or lightly oil a muffin tray.
2. In a small-sized bowl, whisk the egg whites until they are slightly frothy.
3. Mix the egg whites well with the chopped red bell pepper.
4. Fill each muffin tray about three-quarters of the way to the top with the egg and bell pepper mixture.
5. Roast in the preheated oven for 20 minutes or until the egg muffins are set and become slightly golden on top.
6. Before gently removing the muffins from the tray, take them out of the oven and allow them to cool for a few minutes.
7. Store in the fridge for up to 3 days or serve warm.

NUTRITIONAL:
Calories: 25
Protein: 3 g
Fat: 1 g
Carbohydrates: 1 g
Sodium: 15 mg
Potassium: 30 mg
Phosphorus: 10 mg

STRAWBERRY AND PEANUT OATMEAL BOWL

 **PREP TIME:** 5 minutes 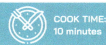 **COOK TIME:** 10 minutes   **SERVINGS:** 1

A creamy and satisfying oatmeal bowl topped with fresh strawberries and a hint of peanut flavor.

INGREDIENTS:

- 1/2 cup rolled oats (40 g)
- 1 cup unsweetened almond milk (240 mL)
- 1/4 cup diced fresh strawberries (40 g)
- 1 teaspoon natural peanut butter (5 g)

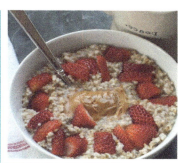

INSTRUCTIONS:

1. In a small-sized saucepan, combine the rolled oats and almond milk. Stir to mix evenly.
2. Put the saucepan on medium heat and bring to a moderate boil, stirring often to prevent the mixture from sticking.
3. Reduce the heat to low and let the oatmeal simmer for 5 to 7 minutes or until the oats become tender and the mixture reaches your desired consistency.
4. Transfer the cooked oatmeal to a serving bowl.
5. Top the oatmeal with the diced strawberries and a drizzle of natural peanut butter.
6. Serve warm, and enjoy immediately.

NUTRITIONAL:
Calories: 170
Protein: 5 g
Fat: 5 g
Carbohydrates: 25 g
Sodium: 50 mg
Potassium: 120 mg
Phosphorus: 60 mg

CUCUMBER AVOCADO WRAP

 **PREP TIME:** 5 minutes   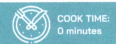 **COOK TIME:** 0 minutes   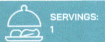 **SERVINGS:** 1

A refreshing and light wrap with creamy avocado, crisp cucumber, and a tangy hint of lemon.

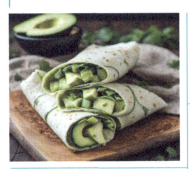

INGREDIENTS:

- 1 low-sodium tortilla (30 g)
- 1 thin slice of avocado (15 g)
- 1/4 cup peeled and thinly sliced cucumber (30 g)
- 1/2 teaspoon lemon juice (2.5 mL)

INSTRUCTIONS:

1. Lay the low-sodium tortilla flat on a clean surface.
2. Place the thin avocado slice on one side of the tortilla and spread it slightly using a spoon or fork.
3. Add the peeled and thinly sliced cucumber on top of the avocado.
4. Drizzle the lemon juice evenly over the cucumber and avocado.
5. Roll the tortilla tightly into a wrap, ensuring the filling is secure.
6. Slice the wrap in half, if desired, and serve immediately.

NUTRITIONAL:

Calories: 90
Protein: 2 g
Fat: 3 g
Carbohydrates: 13 g
Sodium: 35 mg
Potassium: 80 mg
Phosphorus: 20 mg

FRUIT SALAD

 **PREP TIME:** 5 minutes   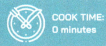 **COOK TIME:** 0 minutes   **SERVINGS:** 2

A vibrant and refreshing mix of kidney-friendly fruits, perfect for a light snack or dessert.

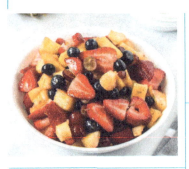

INGREDIENTS:

- 1/4 cup fresh blueberries (40 g)
- 1/4 cup chopped strawberries (40 g)
- 1/2 medium peeled apple, diced (75 g)
- 1/4 cup fresh pineapple chunks (50 g)

INSTRUCTIONS:

1. Rinse the blueberries and strawberries thoroughly under cold water. Pat them dry with a clean towel.
2. Cut the strawberries into tiny pieces after removing the stems.
3. Peel the apple and dice it into bite-sized chunks.
4. Chop the fresh pineapple into similar-sized pieces as the other fruits.
5. In a mixing bowl, combine the blueberries, strawberries, diced apple, and pineapple chunks.
6. Toss gently to mix the fruits evenly.
7. Serve right away or chill in the fridge for a cool treat.

NUTRITIONAL:

Calories: 50
Protein: 0.5 g
Fat: 0.2 g
Carbohydrates: 12 g
Sodium: 2 mg
Potassium: 90 mg
Phosphorus: 15 mg

BREAKFAST MUFFINS

 **PREP TIME:** 10 minutes

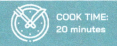 **COOK TIME:** 20 minutes

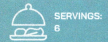 **SERVINGS:** 6

Light and fluffy muffins made with blueberries are perfect for a kidney-friendly breakfast or snack.

INGREDIENTS:

- 1 cup all-purpose flour (120 g)
- 2 egg whites (1/4 cup or 60 mL)
- 2 tablespoons olive oil (30 mL)
- 1/2 cup fresh blueberries (75 g)
- 1 teaspoon baking powder (4 g)
- 1/4 cup water (60 mL)

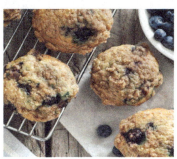

INSTRUCTIONS:

1. Reheat the oven to 350°F (or 175°C) and then gently grease a muffin tray with olive oil or use paper liners.
2. Put the baking powder and all-purpose flour in a mixing basin. To guarantee that the baking powder is dispersed uniformly, thoroughly mix.
3. In another bowl, mix the egg whites, olive oil, and water until smooth.
4. Add the wet components to the dry ingredients, stirring gently until just combined. Do not overmix.
5. Evenly distribute the fresh blueberries throughout the batter by folding them in.
6. Fill each muffin tin cup approximately three-quarters of the way to the top with the batter using a spoon.
7. A toothpick put into the middle of a muffin should come out clean after 18 to 20 minutes of baking in the oven.
8. After taking the muffins out of the oven, let them cool in the muffin tray for five minutes before moving them to a wire rack to finish cooling.

NUTRITIONAL:

Calories: 90
Protein: 2 g
Fat: 3 g
Carbohydrates: 13 g
Sodium: 10 mg
Potassium: 50 mg
Phosphorus: 30 mg

SOUPS

VEGETABLE SOUP

 **PREP TIME:** 10 minutes   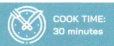 **COOK TIME:** 30 minutes   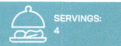 **SERVINGS:** 4

A hearty and nourishing soup packed with kidney-friendly vegetables and warm flavors.

INGREDIENTS:

- 1 medium carrot, diced (70 g)
- 1 medium zucchini, diced (200 g)
- 1/2 cup green beans, chopped (75 g)
- 1 stalk celery, diced (50 g)
- 1/2 small onion, chopped (50 g)
- 1 clove garlic, minced (3 g)
- 1 tablespoon olive oil (15 mL)
- 4 cups low-sodium vegetable broth (1 L)
- 1/4 teaspoon ground black pepper (0.5 g)

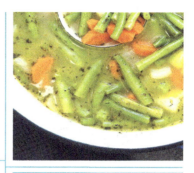

INSTRUCTIONS:

1. Reheat 1 tablespoon olive oil in a large pot on medium-high heat.
2. Add the chopped onion, garlic, celery, and carrots to the pot. Sauté for 5 minutes, stirring occasionally, until the vegetables begin to soften.
3. Stir in the zucchini and green beans. Cook for another 3 to 4 minutes.
4. Pour in the low-sodium vegetable broth and bring the mixture to a boil.
5. Simmer the soup for 20 minutes or until all the veggies are soft, after lowering the heat to low and covering the pot.
6. Add the black pepper and stir well. Adjust seasoning to taste if necessary.
7. Replace the soup from the heat and let it cool slightly before serving.

Calories: 60
Protein: 2 g
Fat: 2 g
Carbohydrates: 8 g
Sodium: 50 mg
Potassium: 120 mg
Phosphorus: 30 mg

NUTRITIONAL:

CHICKEN AND RICE SOUP

 **PREP TIME:** 10 minutes   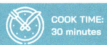 **COOK TIME:** 30 minutes   **SERVINGS:** 4

A comforting and hearty soup with tender chicken, rice, and fresh vegetables.

INGREDIENTS:

- 1 boneless, skinless chicken breast (6 oz / 170 g)
- 1/2 cup uncooked white rice (85 g)
- 1 medium carrot, diced (70 g)
- 1 stalk celery, diced (50 g)
- 1/2 small onion, chopped (50 g)
- 1 clove garlic, minced (3 g)
- 4 cups low-sodium chicken broth (1 L)
- 1 tablespoon fresh parsley, chopped (4 g)

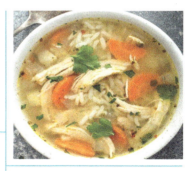

INSTRUCTIONS:

1. In a large pot, bring the low-sodium chicken broth to a gentle boil on medium-high heat.
2. Add the chicken breast to the broth. Cover and cook for 15 minutes or until the chicken is cooked and no longer pink in the center.
3. Replace the chicken breast from the pot and set it aside to cool slightly. Use two forks and shred the chicken into tiny pieces.
4. Add the chopped carrot, celery, onion, and minced garlic to the saucepan while the chicken cools. Let the vegetables simmer for 10 minutes or until tender.
5. Stir in the uncooked white rice. Top the pot and let the rice cook for about 10 minutes or until tender.
6. Add the chicken shreds back to the saucepan and mix everything together. Let the soup simmer for 5 more minutes to heat through.
7. Add the chopped parsley and stir well. Adjust seasoning to taste if necessary.
8. Replace the soup from the heat, and serve warm.

Calories: 120
Protein: 10 g
Fat: 2 g
Carbohydrates: 15 g
Sodium: 50 mg
Potassium: 150 mg
Phosphorus: 90 mg

NUTRITIONAL:

CREAMY CAULIFLOWER SOUP

 **PREP TIME:** 10 minutes   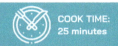 **COOK TIME:** 25 minutes   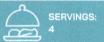 **SERVINGS:** 4

A smooth and comforting soup with the delicate flavor of cauliflower and a touch of thyme.

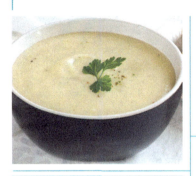

INGREDIENTS:

- 1 head of cauliflower, chopped into florets (600 g)
- 1 cup unsweetened almond milk (240 mL)
- 1 clove garlic, minced (3 g)
- 1 tablespoon olive oil (15 mL)
- 1/2 small onion, chopped (50 g)
- 1/4 teaspoon ground black pepper (0.5 g)
- 1/2 teaspoon fresh thyme leaves (1 g)

INSTRUCTIONS:

1. Reheat the olive oil in a pot over medium heat.
2. Put the onion and minced garlic in the pot. Sauté for 3 to 4 minutes, stirring occasionally, until the onion is softened and translucent.
3. Add the cauliflower florets to the pot and stir to coat them with the oil and aromatics.
4. Pour in 3 cups of water (or enough to cover the cauliflower). The mixture should be brought to a boil over medium heat.
5. Reduce the heat to low, top the pot, and simmer for 15 to 20 minutes or until the cauliflower becomes tender and easily pierced with a fork.
6. Remove the pot from the heat and let the mixture cool slightly. Puree the soup in a handheld blender until it's creamy and smooth.
7. Stir in the almond milk, black pepper, and fresh thyme. Return the pot to low heat and simmer for 5 minutes, stirring occasionally.
8. Serve warm, adjusting spice to taste.

NUTRITIONAL:
Calories: 70
Protein: 2 g
Fat: 3 g
Carbohydrates: 8 g
Sodium: 30 mg
Potassium: 120 mg
Phosphorus: 30 mg

LEMON HERB CHICKEN SOUP

 **PREP TIME:** 10 minutes   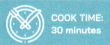 **COOK TIME:** 30 minutes   **SERVINGS:** 4

A light and zesty chicken soup with the freshness of lemon and parsley, perfect for a wholesome meal.

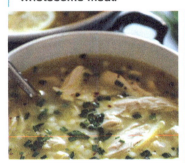

INGREDIENTS:

- 1 boneless, skinless chicken breast (6 oz / 170 g)
- 1/2 cup uncooked white rice (85 g)
- 2 stalks celery, diced (100 g)
- 1 tablespoon lemon juice (15 mL)
- 1 tablespoon fresh parsley, chopped (4 g)
- 4 cups low-sodium chicken broth (1 L)
- 1/4 teaspoon ground black pepper (0.5 g)

INSTRUCTIONS:

1. In a large-sized saucepan on medium-high heat, bring the low-sodium chicken broth to a boil.
2. Add the chicken breast to the pot. Cover and simmer for 15 minutes or until the chicken is fully cooked and tender.
3. Replace the chicken breast from the pot and set it aside to cool slightly. Use two forks and shred the chicken into small pieces.
4. Put the diced celery in the pot and let it simmer for 5 minutes.
5. Stir in the uncooked white rice and let the soup stew for an additional 10 minutes or until the rice is tender.
6. Add the chicken shreds back to the saucepan and mix everything together.
7. Add the lemon juice, chopped parsley, and black pepper. Stir well and let the soup simmer for 2 more minutes.
8. Remove from heat and serve warm.

NUTRITIONAL:
Calories: 120
Protein: 12 g
Fat: 1 g
Carbohydrates: 15 g
Sodium: 50 mg
Potassium: 150 mg
Phosphorus: 90 mg

ZUCCHINI AND HERB SOUP

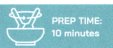 **PREP TIME:** 10 minutes
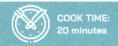 **COOK TIME:** 20 minutes
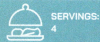 **SERVINGS:** 4

A light and flavorful soup featuring tender zucchini and fresh herbs.

INGREDIENTS:

- 2 medium zucchini, diced (400 g)
- 2 cloves garlic, minced (6 g)
- 1 tablespoon olive oil (15 mL)
- 4 cups low-sodium vegetable broth (1 L)
- 1 tablespoon fresh parsley, chopped (4 g)
- 1/2 teaspoon fresh thyme leaves (1 g)

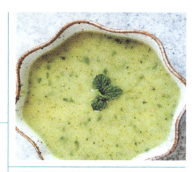

INSTRUCTIONS:

1. Reheat the olive oil in a pot over medium heat.
2. Put the minced garlic and sauté for 1 to 2 minutes until fragrant, being careful not to let it burn.
3. Stir in the diced zucchini and cook for 5 minutes, stirring occasionally, until the zucchini starts to soften.
4. Add the veggie broth with low sodium and bring to a boil over medium heat.
5. Reduce the heat to low, top the pot, and let the soup stew for 15 minutes or until the zucchini is tender.
6. Replace the pot from the heat. Take a blender and puree the soup until smooth. Alternatively, remove the soup from a blender in batches.
7. Stir in the fresh parsley and thyme, mixing well. Adjust seasoning with additional black pepper if desired.
8. Serve warm, and season with a sprinkle of parsley if preferred

Calories: 60
Protein: 1.5 g
Fat: 2 g
Carbohydrates: 8 g
Sodium: 35 mg
Potassium: 140 mg
Phosphorus: 20 mg

NUTRITIONAL:

CABBAGE AND CARROT SOUP

 **PREP TIME:** 10 minutes
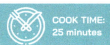 **COOK TIME:** 25 minutes
 SERVINGS: 4

With the natural sweetness of carrots and the crunch of cabbage, this soup is substantial and comforting.

INGREDIENTS:

- 2 cups chopped cabbage (150 g)
- 1 medium carrot, diced (70 g)
- 1/2 medium onion, finely chopped (50 g)
- 1 clove garlic, minced (3 g)
- 1 tablespoon olive oil (15 mL)
- 4 cups low-sodium vegetable broth (1 L)
- 1/4 teaspoon ground black pepper (0.5 g)

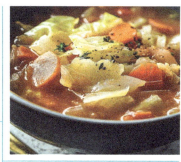

INSTRUCTIONS:

1. Reheat the olive oil in a pot over medium heat.
2. Put the chopped onion and garlic in the pot and sauté for 2 to 3 minutes until the onion is softened and fragrant.
3. Stir in the diced carrot and cook for another 3 minutes, stirring occasionally.
4. Put the chopped cabbage in the pot and mix well with the other vegetables. Cook for 2 minutes to slightly wilt the cabbage.
5. Add the veggie broth with low sodium and bring to a boil over medium heat.
6. Reduce the heat to low, top the pot, and let the soup boil for 15 minutes or until the vegetables are tender.
7. Add the ground black pepper and stir well. Adjust seasoning to taste if necessary.
8. Remove the soup from the heat and serve warm.

Calories: 50
Protein: 1 g
Fat: 2 g
Carbohydrates: 7 g
Sodium: 35 mg
Potassium: 120 mg
Phosphorus: 20 mg

NUTRITIONAL:

CREAMY CARROT GINGER SOUP

 **PREP TIME:** 10 minutes 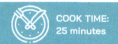 **COOK TIME:** 25 minutes 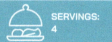 **SERVINGS:** 4

A smooth and aromatic soup with the natural sweetness of carrots and a hint of fresh ginger.

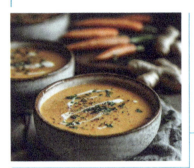

INGREDIENTS:

- 4 medium carrots, chopped (300 g)
- 1 teaspoon freshly grated ginger (2 g)
- 1/2 medium onion, finely chopped (50 g)
- 1 tablespoon olive oil (15 mL)
- 1 cup unsweetened almond milk (240 mL)
- 2 cups water (480 mL)
- 1/4 teaspoon ground black pepper (0.5 g)

INSTRUCTIONS:

1. Reheat the olive oil in a pot over medium heat.
2. Add the chopped onion and sauté for 2 to 3 minutes until softened and translucent.
3. Stir in the chopped carrots and grated ginger. Cook for 4 minutes, stirring occasionally.
4. Add the water and bring to a boil over medium heat.
5. Reduce the heat to low, top the pot, and let the soup boil for 15 to 20 minutes or until the carrots are tender and easily pierced with a fork.
6. Remove the pot from heat and let the mixture cool slightly. Puree the soup in a handheld blender until it's smooth.
7. Stir in the unsweetened almond milk and ground black pepper. Return the pot to low heat and cook for 5 minutes, stirring occasionally.
8. Adjust seasoning as needed and serve warm.

NUTRITIONAL:
Calories: 60
Protein: 1 g
Fat: 2 g
Carbohydrates: 9 g
Sodium: 20 mg
Potassium: 130 mg
Phosphorus: 20 mg

PUMPKIN SOUP

 PREP TIME: 10 minutes 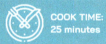 **COOK TIME:** 25 minutes **SERVINGS:** 4

A creamy and lightly spiced soup highlighting the natural sweetness of pumpkin and a hint of nutmeg.

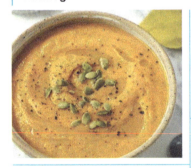

INGREDIENTS:

- 2 cups diced fresh pumpkin (low-potassium variety, about 300 g)
- 1 clove garlic, minced (3 g)
- 1 cup unsweetened almond milk (240 mL)
- 1 tablespoon olive oil (15 mL)
- 2 cups water (480 mL)
- 1/4 teaspoon ground black pepper (0.5 g)
- 1/8 teaspoon ground nutmeg (0.25 g)

INSTRUCTIONS:

1. Reheat the olive oil in a pot over medium heat.
2. Put the chopped onion and garlic in the pot and sauté for 1 to 2 minutes until the onion is fragrant.
3. Coat the diced pumpkin with the olive oil and garlic by stirring in the mixture. Saute for three to four minutes, tossing every so often.
4. Then, add the water and boil it over medium-high heat.
5. For about fifteen to twenty minutes, or until the pumpkin is soft and readily punctured with a fork, bring the soup to a simmer over low heat, covered.
6. Put the saucepan off the heat and give the ingredients a little time to cool. To make a smooth puree, either use a handheld blender or transfer the soup to a processor in phases.
7. Stir in the unsweetened almond milk, ground black pepper, and nutmeg. Return the soup to low heat and simmer for 5 minutes, stirring occasionally.
8. Adjust seasoning as desired and serve warm.

NUTRITIONAL:
Calories: 70
Protein: 1 g
Fat: 3 g
Carbohydrates: 10 g
Sodium: 15 mg
Potassium: 120 mg
Phosphorus: 20 mg

BARLEY AND VEGETABLE SOUP

 **PREP TIME:** 10 minutes   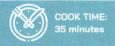 **COOK TIME:** 35 minutes   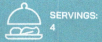 **SERVINGS:** 4

A hearty and wholesome soup with tender barley and fresh vegetables, perfect for a comforting meal.

INGREDIENTS:

- 1/4 cup uncooked barley (50 g)
- 1 medium carrot, diced (70 g)
- 1 stalk celery, diced (50 g)
- 1/2 medium onion, finely chopped (50 g)
- 1 clove garlic, minced (3 g)
- 1 tablespoon olive oil (15 mL)
- 4 cups low-sodium vegetable broth (1 L)
- 1 tablespoon fresh parsley, chopped (4 g)

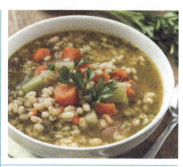

INSTRUCTIONS:

1. Reheat the olive oil in a pot over medium heat.
2. Put the chopped onion and garlic in the pot and sauté for 2 to 3 minutes until the onion is softened and fragrant.
3. Add the celery and carrots that have been diced, and continue cooking for another three or four minutes, stirring regularly.
4. Coat the barley with the oil and veggies by adding them to the pot and stirring them. Cook for 1 to 2 minutes.
5. Over medium-high heat, add the vegetable broth with low sodium and bring to a boil.
6. As soon as the barley reaches the desired tenderness, reduce the heat to a low setting, wrap around the pot, and allow the soup to simmer for thirty minutes.
7. Mix the chopped parsley thoroughly after stirring it. Adjust seasoning with additional black pepper if desired.
8. Serve warm and garnish with more parsley, if preferred.

NUTRITIONAL:
Calories: 80
Protein: 2 g
Fat: 2 g
Carbohydrates: 13 g
Sodium: 40 mg
Potassium: 100 mg
Phosphorus: 30 mg

PARSLEY POTATO SOUP

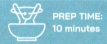 **PREP TIME:** 10 minutes   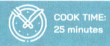 **COOK TIME:** 25 minutes   **SERVINGS:** 4

A simple and comforting soup with creamy potatoes and the freshness of parsley.

INGREDIENTS:

- 1 small white potato, diced (100 g)
- 1/2 medium onion, finely chopped (50 g)
- 1 clove garlic, minced (3 g)
- 1 tablespoon olive oil (15 mL)
- 4 cups low-sodium chicken broth (1 L)
- 2 tablespoons fresh parsley, chopped (8 g)
- 1/4 teaspoon ground black pepper (0.5 g)

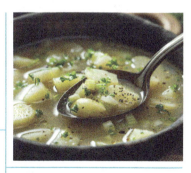

INSTRUCTIONS:

1. Reheat the olive oil in a pot over medium heat.
2. Put the chopped onion and garlic in the pot and sauté for 2 to 3 minutes until the onion is softened and fragrant.
3. Stir in the diced potato and cook for another 2 to 3 minutes, stirring occasionally.
4. After adding the chicken broth with a low sodium content, bring the mixture to a boil over medium-high heat after pouring it in.
5. After the potato is soft and readily punctured with a fork, bring the soup to a simmer over low heat, cover, and cook it for 20 minutes.
6. For a smoother consistency, purée the soup using an immersion blender. If you like a more rustic texture, leave it lumpy.
7. Stir in the chopped parsley and black pepper, mixing well. Let the soup simmer for 2 more minutes.
8. After taking it off the stove, serve it warm with extra parsley on top if you like.

NUTRITIONAL:
Calories: 60
Protein: 2 g
Fat: 2 g
Carbohydrates: 9 g
Sodium: 40 mg
Potassium: 110 mg
Phosphorus: 30 mg

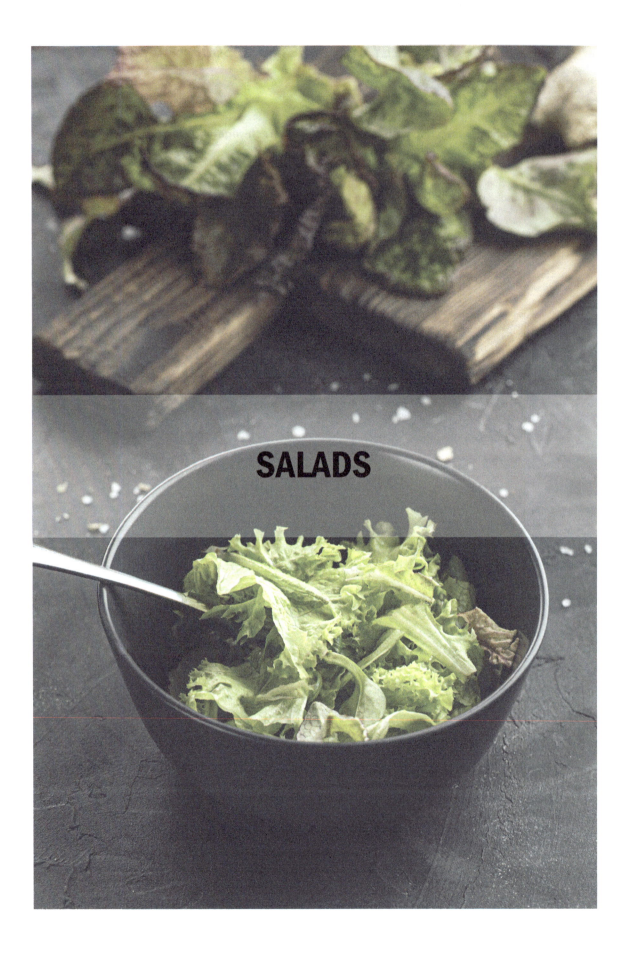

SALADS

CUCUMBER AND HERB SALAD

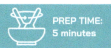 **PREP TIME:** 5 minutes 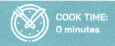 **COOK TIME:** 0 minutes 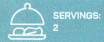 **SERVINGS:** 2

A refreshing and light salad with crisp cucumber and fresh parsley.

INGREDIENTS:

- 1 large cucumber, peeled and thinly sliced (200 g)
- 2 tablespoons fresh parsley, chopped (8 g)
- 1 teaspoon olive oil (5 mL)
- 1 teaspoon lemon juice (5 mL)
- 1/8 teaspoon ground black pepper (0.3 g)

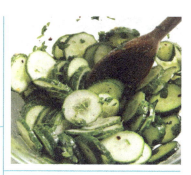

INSTRUCTIONS:

1. Peel the cucumber and slice it thinly into rounds. Place the slices in a mixing bowl.
2. Combine the cucumber and chopped parsley in a bowl.
3. After mixing the parsley and cucumber, drizzle with some olive oil and squeeze the lemon juice.
4. Sprinkle the ground black pepper evenly over the salad.
5. Toss the ingredients gently to ensure everything is well coated.
6. Quickly transfer the salad to plates for serving.

NUTRITIONAL:
Calories: 30
Protein: 1 g
Fat: 1.5 g
Carbohydrates: 3 g
Sodium: 5 mg
Potassium: 100 mg
Phosphorus: 10 mg

APPLE AND CABBAGE SLAW

 **PREP TIME:** 10 minutes 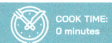 **COOK TIME:** 0 minutes   **SERVINGS:** 4

A crisp and tangy slaw with the sweetness of apple and the crunch of cabbage.

INGREDIENTS:

- 2 cups shredded cabbage (150 g)
- 1 medium peeled apple, julienned (150 g)
- 1 tablespoon apple cider vinegar (15 mL)
- 1 tablespoon olive oil (15 mL)
- 1/4 teaspoon ground black pepper (0.5 g)

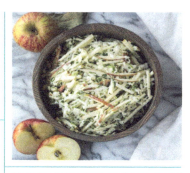

INSTRUCTIONS:

1. In a big mixing basin, add the shredded cabbage.
2. Peel the apple and cut it into thin julienne strips. Add the apple to the bowl with the cabbage.
3. Blend the ground black pepper, olive oil, and the vinegar made from apple cider in a small bowl and whisk to blend.
4. Pour the dressing over the cabbage and apple mixture.
5. Gently combine all the ingredients, making sure to coat them uniformly with the dressing.
6. Feel free to serve it right away or give it a quick 15 minutes in the fridge for a crunchier texture.

NUTRITIONAL:
Calories: 50
Protein: 1 g
Fat: 3 g
Carbohydrates: 6 g
Sodium: 5 mg
Potassium: 80 mg
Phosphorus: 15 mg

CARROT AND ZUCCHINI RIBBON SALAD

 PREP TIME: 10 minutes

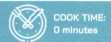 COOK TIME: 0 minutes

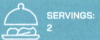 SERVINGS: 2

A vibrant and refreshing salad with delicate ribbons of carrot and zucchini dressed with lemon and dill.

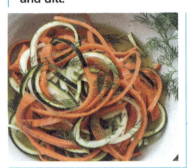

INGREDIENTS:

- 1 medium carrot, shredded or cut into ribbons (70 g)
- 1 medium zucchini, cut into ribbons (150 g)
- 1 teaspoon olive oil (5 mL)
- 1 teaspoon lemon juice (5 mL)
- 1 tablespoon fresh dill, chopped (4 g)

INSTRUCTIONS:

1. After the carrot is washed and peeled, you may either chop it into thin ribbons or use a vegetable peeler.
2. After you give the zucchini a good wash, slice it lengthwise into thin ribbons using a vegetable peeler.
3. Place the carrot and zucchini ribbons in a mixing bowl.
4. Apply a drizzle of olive oil and lemon juice onto the vegetables.
5. Sprinkle the fresh dill over the mixture.
6. Coat the veggies uniformly with the dressing and lightly toss to incorporate the ingredients.
7. Serve immediately or chill briefly before serving for enhanced flavor.

NUTRITIONAL:
Calories: 40
Protein: 1 g
Fat: 2 g
Carbohydrates: 4 g
Sodium: 5 mg
Potassium: 100 mg
Phosphorus: 10 mg

BERRY SPINACH SALAD

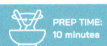 PREP TIME: 10 minutes

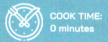 COOK TIME: 0 minutes

 SERVINGS: 2

A delightful and refreshing salad with sweet berries and tender baby spinach.

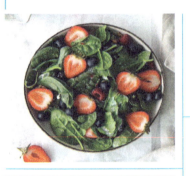

INGREDIENTS:

- 1 cup baby spinach leaves (30 g)
- 1/4 cup sliced strawberries (40 g)
- 1/4 cup fresh blueberries (40 g)
- 1 teaspoon olive oil (5 mL)
- 1 teaspoon balsamic vinegar (5 mL)

INSTRUCTIONS:

1. Rinse the baby spinach, strawberries, and blueberries thoroughly under cold water. Pat them dry with a clean towel.
2. Place the baby spinach in a mixing bowl.
3. Toss the spinach with the sliced strawberries and blueberries in a bowl.
4. Apply a drizzle of olive oil and balsamic vinegar onto the salad components.
5. Toss gently to coat the spinach and berries with the dressing.
6. Serve immediately and enjoy.

NUTRITIONAL:
Calories: 40
Protein: 1 g
Fat: 2 g
Carbohydrates: 5 g
Sodium: 5 mg
Potassium: 80 mg
Phosphorus: 15 mg

QUINOA AND CUCUMBER SALAD

 **PREP TIME:** 10 minutes

 **COOK TIME:** 15 minutes

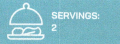 **SERVINGS:** 2

A refreshing and light salad with protein-rich quinoa, crisp cucumber, and fresh parsley.

INGREDIENTS:

- 1/2 cup cooked quinoa (85 g)
- 1/2 cup peeled and diced cucumber (75 g)
- 1 teaspoon olive oil (5 mL)
- 1 tablespoon fresh parsley, chopped (4 g)
- 1 teaspoon lemon juice (5 mL)

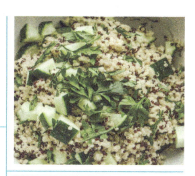

INSTRUCTIONS:

1. If you haven't done so already, cook the quinoa per the package directions. Let it cool to room temperature.
2. Peel the cucumber and dice it into small cubes. Place it in a mixing bowl.
3. Add the cooked quinoa and chopped parsley to the bowl with the cucumber.
4. Apply a drizzle of olive oil and lemon juice onto the mixture.
5. Gently toss to uniformly mix all ingredients.
6. Put it in the fridge for 15 minutes to cool down, or serve it right away if you prefer a colder salad.

Calories: 60
Protein: 2 g
Fat: 2 g
Carbohydrates: 8 g
Sodium: 5 mg
Potassium: 40 mg
Phosphorus: 25 mg

NUTRITIONAL:

CAULIFLOWER «RICE» SALAD

 **PREP TIME:** 10 minutes

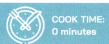 **COOK TIME:** 0 minutes

 SERVINGS: 2

A light and flavorful salad with riced cauliflower and fresh, vibrant vegetables.

INGREDIENTS:

- 1 cup riced cauliflower (100 g)
- 1/4 cup diced red bell pepper (40 g)
- 1 tablespoon fresh parsley, chopped (4 g)
- 1 teaspoon olive oil (5 mL)
- 1 teaspoon lemon juice (5 mL)

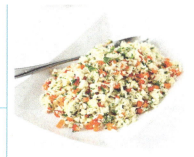

INSTRUCTIONS:

1. If using fresh cauliflower, pulse small florets in a food processor until they resemble rice. Alternatively, use pre-riced cauliflower.
2. Place the riced cauliflower in a mixing bowl.
3. Incorporate the chopped parsley and diced red bell pepper into the basin containing the cauliflower.
4. Apply a drizzle of olive oil and lemon juice onto the mixture.
5. Toss gently to mix everything evenly and coat with the dressing.
6. Serve promptly or refrigerate for a refreshing dish.

Calories: 40
Protein: 1.5 g
Fat: 2 g
Carbohydrates: 4 g
Sodium: 5 mg
Potassium: 60 mg
Phosphorus: 15 mg

NUTRITIONAL:

GREEN BEAN AND TOMATO SALAD

 **PREP TIME:** 10 minutes   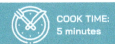 **COOK TIME:** 5 minutes   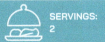 **SERVINGS:** 2

A crisp and tangy salad featuring steamed green beans and juicy cherry tomatoes.

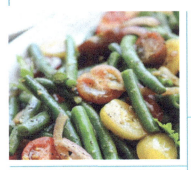

INGREDIENTS:

- 1 cup steamed green beans, trimmed and cut into bite-sized pieces (100 g)
- 75 grams of halved cherry tomatoes (1/2 cup)
- 1 teaspoon olive oil (5 mL)
- 1 teaspoon balsamic vinegar (5 mL)
- 1/8 teaspoon ground black pepper (0.3 g)

INSTRUCTIONS:

1. Steam the green beans until tender-crisp, about 3 to 5 minutes. Let them cool slightly.
2. Place the steamed green beans and halved cherry tomatoes in a mixing bowl.
3. Apply a drizzle of olive oil and lemon juice over the vegetables.
4. Sprinkle with ground black pepper.
5. Gently toss to uniformly coat the vegetables with the dressing.
6. Serve promptly or refrigerate for a chilled salad.

NUTRITIONAL:
Calories: 50
Protein: 1.5 g
Fat: 2 g
Carbohydrates: 6 g
Sodium: 5 mg
Potassium: 100 mg
Phosphorus: 20 mg

ZUCCHINI AND RED BELL PEPPER SALAD

 **PREP TIME:** 10 minutes   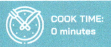 **COOK TIME:** 0 minutes   **SERVINGS:** 2

A fresh and colorful salad featuring tender zucchini slices and sweet red bell pepper with a hint of basil.

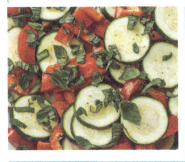

INGREDIENTS:

- 1 medium zucchini, thinly sliced (150 g)
- 1/4 cup diced red bell pepper (40 g)
- 1 teaspoon olive oil (5 mL)
- 1 teaspoon lemon juice (5 mL)
- 1 tablespoon fresh basil, chopped (4 g)

INSTRUCTIONS:

1. Wash the zucchini and use a mandoline or knife to thinly slice it into rounds.
2. Toss the zucchini slices and the red bell pepper cubes into a mixing dish.
3. Apply a drizzle of olive oil and lemon juice over the vegetables.
4. Sprinkle the chopped fresh basil over the salad.
5. Toss gently to coat the zucchini and bell pepper evenly with the dressing.
6. Serve promptly or refrigerate for a more invigorating flavor.

NUTRITIONAL:
Calories: 35
Protein: 1 g
Fat: 2 g
Carbohydrates: 4 g
Sodium: 5 mg
Potassium: 100 mg
Phosphorus: 15 mg

CABBAGE AND RADISH SALAD

 **PREP TIME:** 10 minutes   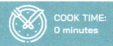 **COOK TIME:** 0 minutes   **SERVINGS:** 2

A crisp and tangy salad with crunchy cabbage and zesty radishes.

INGREDIENTS:

- 1 cup shredded cabbage (75 g)
- 1/2 cup thinly sliced radish (50 g)
- 1 teaspoon olive oil (5 mL)
- 1 teaspoon apple cider vinegar (5 mL)
- 1/8 teaspoon ground black pepper (0.3 g)

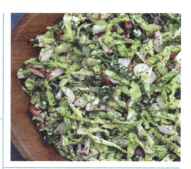

INSTRUCTIONS:

1. Transfer the shredded cabbage to a mixing dish.
2. Add the thinly sliced radishes to the bowl.
3. Apply a drizzle of olive oil and apple cider vinegar over the vegetables.
4. Sprinkle the ground black pepper over the salad.
5. Gently toss to uniformly mix all ingredients.
6. For the best flavor, serve right away or refrigerate for 10 minutes.

Calories: 25
Protein: 1 g
Fat: 1 g
Carbohydrates: 3 g
Sodium: 5 mg
Potassium: 70 mg
Phosphorus: 10 mg

NUTRITIONAL:

PARSLEY POTATO SALAD

 **PREP TIME:** 10 minutes   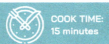 **COOK TIME:** 15 minutes   **SERVINGS:** 2

A simple and flavorful salad with tender potatoes, fresh parsley, and a hint of lemon.

INGREDIENTS:

- 1 small white potato, diced (100 g)
- 1 teaspoon olive oil (5 mL)
- 1 tablespoon fresh parsley, chopped (4 g)
- 1 teaspoon lemon juice (5 mL)
- 1/8 teaspoon ground black pepper (0.3 g)

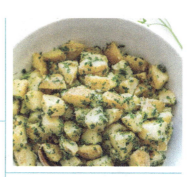

INSTRUCTIONS:

1. Peel and dice the small white potato into bite-sized cubes.
2. Place the diced potato in a pot of water and bring it to a boil. Cook for 10 to 12 minutes or until the potato is tender but not mushy.
3. Drain the cooked potato and let it cool to room temperature.
4. Juice the lemon and add the ground black pepper to the olive oil in a mixing bowl. Stir to mix.
5. Add the cooled potato and chopped parsley to the bowl. Toss gently to coat the potatoes evenly with the dressing.
6. Put it in the fridge for 15 minutes to cool down, or serve it right away if you prefer a colder salad.

Calories: 60
Protein: 1 g
Fat: 2 g
Carbohydrates: 9 g
Sodium: 5 mg
Potassium: 80 mg
Phosphorus: 20 mg

NUTRITIONAL:

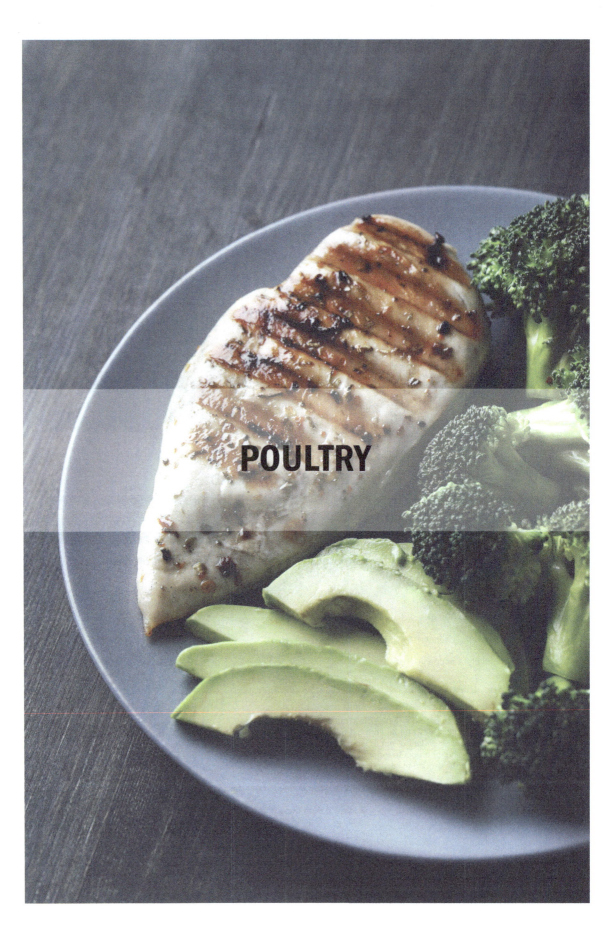

POULTRY

LEMON HERB CHICKEN BREAST

 **PREP TIME:** 10 minutes

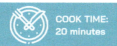 **COOK TIME:** 20 minutes

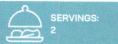 **SERVINGS:** 2

With a zesty marinade of lemon and herbs, this meal of chicken is moist and tasty.

INGREDIENTS:

- 2 boneless, skinless chicken breasts (5 oz / 140 g each)
- 1 tablespoon olive oil (15 mL)
- 1 clove garlic, minced (3 g)
- 1 tablespoon lemon juice (15 mL)
- 1 tablespoon fresh parsley, chopped (4 g)
- 1/4 teaspoon ground black pepper (0.5 g)

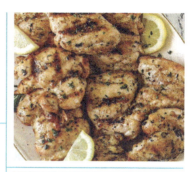

INSTRUCTIONS:

1. Start the oven to 375°F (190°C) or grill the meat in a pan set over medium heat.
2. To prepare the marinade, place the minced garlic, olive oil, lemon juice, chopped parsley, and black pepper in a small bowl.
3. Rub the marinade evenly over both chicken breasts, ensuring they are well coated.
4. To bake, put the chicken breasts in a baking dish and bake for 18 to 20 minutes or until the chicken hits 165°F (74°C) on the inside. If grilling, cook for 6-7 minutes on each side.
5. After taking the chicken out of the oven or grill, let it rest for five minutes so that the fluids can be preserved.
6. Place on a warm platter and, if wanted, sprinkle with more chopped parsley.

Calories: 220
Protein: 32 g
Fat: 9 g
Carbohydrates: 1 g
Sodium: 60 mg
Potassium: 320 mg
Phosphorus: 250 mg

NUTRITIONAL:

GARLIC ROSEMARY ROASTED CHICKEN

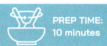 **PREP TIME:** 10 minutes

 **COOK TIME:** 30 minutes

 SERVINGS: 2

A savory and aromatic roasted chicken dish infused with garlic and fresh rosemary.

INGREDIENTS:

- 4 chicken thighs, skin removed (4 oz / 115 g each)
- 1 tablespoon olive oil (15 mL)
- 2 cloves garlic, minced (6 g)
- 1 teaspoon fresh rosemary, chopped (2 g)
- 1/4 teaspoon ground black pepper (0.5 g)

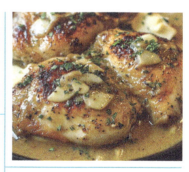

INSTRUCTIONS:

1. Start the oven to 400°F (200°C).
2. To make the marinade, combine some olive oil, ground black pepper, chopped rosemary, and minced garlic in a small bowl.
3. Rub the marinade evenly over the chicken thighs, ensuring all sides are coated.
4. Arrange the chicken thighs in a roasting pan or baking dish in a single layer.
5. After 25 to 30 minutes in a warmed oven or until the chicken gets an internal temperature of 165°F (74°C) and the skin is golden brown, remove from oven.
6. After 5 minutes of cooling, take the chicken out of the oven and set it aside to enjoy.

Calories: 250
Protein: 30 g
Fat: 13 g
Carbohydrates: 1 g
Sodium: 70 mg
Potassium: 320 mg
Phosphorus: 250 mg

NUTRITIONAL:

BAKED CHICKEN WITH ZUCCHINI

 **PREP TIME:** 10 minutes   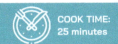 **COOK TIME:** 25 minutes   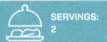 **SERVINGS:** 2

A simple and nutritious dish with tender chicken and roasted zucchini, enhanced with garlic and thyme.

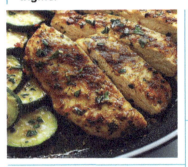

INGREDIENTS:

- 2 boneless, skinless chicken breasts (5 oz / 140 g each)
- 1 medium zucchini, sliced into rounds (200 g)
- 1 tablespoon olive oil (15 mL)
- 1 clove garlic, minced (3 g)
- 1/2 teaspoon dried thyme (1 g)
- 1/4 teaspoon ground black pepper (0.5 g)

INSTRUCTIONS:

1. Start the oven to 375°F (190°C).
2. Whisk together the olive oil, black pepper, dried thyme, and some minced garlic in a small bowl to make the marinade.
3. Place the chicken breasts and zucchini slices in a baking dish.
4. Drizzle the marinade over the chicken and zucchini, ensuring everything is evenly coated.
5. After 20 to 25 minutes in a warmed oven or until the chicken gets an internal temperature of 165°F (74°C) and the skin is golden brown, remove from oven.
6. After 5 minutes of cooling, take the chicken out of the oven and set it aside to enjoy.
7. Serve warm, pairing the chicken with the roasted zucchini.

NUTRITIONAL:
Calories: 200
Protein: 30 g
Fat: 8 g
Carbohydrates: 3 g
Sodium: 55 mg
Potassium: 400 mg
Phosphorus: 250 mg

HONEY MUSTARD GRILLED CHICKEN

 PREP TIME: 10 minutes   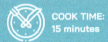 **COOK TIME:** 15 minutes   **SERVINGS:** 2

A sweet and tangy grilled chicken dish with a flavorful honey mustard glaze.

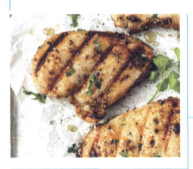

INGREDIENTS:

- 2 boneless, skinless chicken breasts (5 oz / 140 g each)
- 1 tablespoon honey (15 mL)
- 1 tablespoon Dijon mustard (15 mL)
- 1 teaspoon olive oil (5 mL)
- 1/4 teaspoon ground black pepper (0.5 g)

INSTRUCTIONS:

1. In a small bowl, whisk together the honey, Dijon mustard, olive oil, and ground black pepper to make the marinade.
2. The marinade should be poured over the chicken breasts after they have been placed in a shallow dish or a plastic bag that can be sealed back up. Ensure the chicken is evenly coated. Marinate in the refrigerator for at least 15 minutes.
3. Put a grill or pan on high heat to get it ready for cooking.
4. Let the marinade drain off the chicken before removing it. Discard the leftover marinade.
5. After getting the internal temperature to 165°F (74°C), grill the chicken for about 7 or 8 minutes per side.
6. Let the chicken rest for 5 minutes after removing it from the grill.
7. Serve warm, optionally garnished with fresh parsley or a drizzle of honey mustard sauce.

NUTRITIONAL:
Calories: 220
Protein: 30 g
Fat: 5 g
Carbohydrates: 9 g
Sodium: 70 mg
Potassium: 320 mg
Phosphorus: 250 mg

TURKEY AND GREEN BEAN STIR-FRY

 **PREP TIME:** 10 minutes    **COOK TIME:** 15 minutes   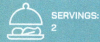 **SERVINGS:** 2

A quick and healthy stir-fry with tender turkey breast and crisp green beans, enhanced with garlic and lemon.

INGREDIENTS:

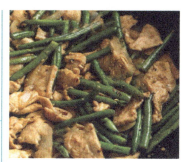

- 8 oz turkey breast, cut into thin strips (225 g)
- one cup (100 g) of green beans, trimmed and chopped into little pieces
- 1 tablespoon olive oil (15 mL)
- 1 clove garlic, minced (3 g)
- 1 teaspoon lemon juice (5 mL)
- 1/4 teaspoon ground black pepper (0.5 g)

INSTRUCTIONS:

1. On medium heat, in a big nonstick skillet, heat half of the olive oil.
2. Toss in the turkey strips and sear them for four to five minutes, stirring once or twice, or until they are browned and cooked through. Lay the turkey aside after taking it out of the pan.
3. Heat up the skillet and add the rest of the olive oil. Toss in the green beans and sauté for 3-4 minutes until they begin to soften.
4. While the green beans and minced garlic are cooking in a skillet, cook for another minute, stirring often.
5. After the turkey has cooked, add it back to the pan and mix it with the green beans.
6. Apply the drizzle of lemon juice over the stir-fry and sprinkle with ground black pepper. Stir well to coat evenly.
7. Cook for 1-2 more minutes to heat everything through.
8. Remove from the heat and serve warm.

NUTRITIONAL:
Calories: 200
Protein: 30 g
Fat: 7 g
Carbohydrates: 3 g
Sodium: 40 mg
Potassium: 300 mg
Phosphorus: 220 mg

CURRY-SPICED CHICKEN THIGHS

 **PREP TIME:** 10 minutes   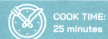 **COOK TIME:** 25 minutes   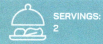 **SERVINGS:** 2

Aromatic and flavorful chicken thighs infused with warm curry spices and a hint of lemon.

INGREDIENTS:

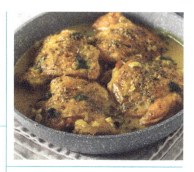

- 4 chicken thighs, skin removed (4 oz / 115 g each)
- 1 tablespoon olive oil (15 mL)
- 1 teaspoon curry powder (2 g)
- 1 clove garlic, minced (3 g)
- 1 teaspoon lemon juice (5 mL)
- 1/4 teaspoon ground black pepper (0.5 g)

INSTRUCTIONS:

1. Whisk together the marinade ingredients (olive oil, curry powder, minced garlic, lemon juice, and black pepper) in a small bowl.
2. In the shallow dish or a plastic bag that can be sealed, lay the chicken thighs. After you've covered the chicken thoroughly, pour the marinade over it. For a minimum of fifteen minutes, marinate it in the fridge.
3. Start the oven to 400°F (200°C) or grill the meat in a pan set over medium heat.
4. Let any extra marinade drain off the chicken thighs before removing them. Throw out the marinade that isn't needed.
5. Put the chicken thighs on a baking dish and roast them for 20-25 minutes, or until they reach an internal temperature of 165°F (74°C), if you want to bake them. If grilling, cook the chicken thighs for 6-7 minutes per side until fully cooked.
6. Give the chicken 5 minutes to rest before cutting it.
7. Serve warm, optionally garnished with fresh parsley or a wedge of lemon.

NUTRITIONAL:
Calories: 260
Protein: 32 g
Fat: 12 g
Carbohydrates: 1 g
Sodium: 70 mg
Potassium: 320 mg
Phosphorus: 250 mg

HERB-CRUSTED CHICKEN TENDERS

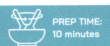 **PREP TIME:** 10 minutes   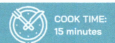 **COOK TIME:** 15 minutes   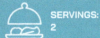 **SERVINGS:** 2

Crispy and flavorful chicken tenders coated with a savory herb blend.

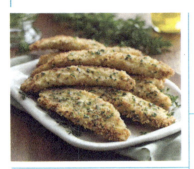

INGREDIENTS:

- 8 oz chicken breast, cut into strips (225 g)
- 1 tablespoon olive oil (15 mL)
- 1 teaspoon dried parsley (2 g)
- 1/2 teaspoon garlic powder (1 g)
- 1/4 teaspoon ground black pepper (0.5 g)

INSTRUCTIONS:

1. Start the oven to 400°F (200°C) or grill the meat in a pan set over medium heat.
2. Herb blend: In a small bowl, mix dried parsley, garlic powder, and black pepper.
3. Brush the chicken breast strips with olive oil on all sides.
4. Coat the chicken strips evenly with the herb blend, pressing gently to adhere.
5. For baking, arrange the chicken tenders on a parchment-lined baking sheet and bake for 12-15 minutes, turning halfway, until fully cooked and the internal temperature is 165°F (74°C).
6. If grilling, cook the chicken tenders for 6-7 minutes per side until they are golden brown and fully cooked.
7. Remove from heat and let the tenders rest for 3 minutes before serving.

NUTRITIONAL:
Calories: 180
Protein: 30 g
Fat: 6 g
Carbohydrates: 1 g
Sodium: 50 mg
Potassium: 300 mg
Phosphorus: 220 mg

TURKEY WITH CAULIFLOWER RICE

 **PREP TIME:** 10 minutes   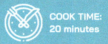 **COOK TIME:** 20 minutes   **SERVINGS:** 2

A light and wholesome dish featuring tender turkey breast and savory cauliflower rice.

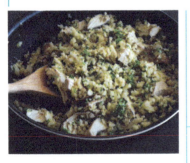

INGREDIENTS:

- 8 oz turkey breast, cut into bite-sized pieces (225 g)
- 2 cups riced cauliflower (200 g)
- 1 tablespoon olive oil (15 mL)
- 1 clove garlic, minced (3 g)
- 1 tablespoon fresh parsley, chopped (4 g)
- 1/4 teaspoon ground black pepper (0.5 g)

INSTRUCTIONS:

1. A big nonstick skillet set over medium heat should be used to heat half of the olive oil.
2. Toss in the turkey breasts and brown them in a skillet over medium heat, tossing periodically, for about 6 to 8 minutes, or until done. Lay the turkey aside after taking it out of the pan.
3. Put the minced garlic and more olive oil into the same pan. To release the aroma, sauté for 1 minute.
4. Bring the riced cauliflower to a simmer in a pan over medium heat, stirring regularly, for 5 to 7 minutes, or until softened.
5. Stir the cooked turkey back into the skillet with the cauliflower rice.
6. Add the chopped parsley and black pepper, mixing well to combine all ingredients.
7. Just give it a quick extra minute or two to heat everything up.
8. Serve warm and enjoy.

NUTRITIONAL:
Calories: 180
Protein: 30 g
Fat: 5 g
Carbohydrates: 4 g
Sodium: 30 mg
Potassium: 250 mg
Phosphorus: 220 mg

STUFFED CHICKEN BREAST

 **PREP TIME:** 15 minutes   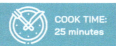 **COOK TIME:** 25 minutes   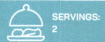 **SERVINGS:** 2

A flavorful and healthy stuffed chicken breast filled with zucchini, red bell pepper, and garlic.

INGREDIENTS:

- 2 boneless, skinless chicken breasts (5 oz / 140 g each)
- 1/4 cup finely diced zucchini (40 g)
- 40 g finely chopped red bell pepper
- 1 clove garlic, minced (3 g)
- 1 tablespoon olive oil (15 mL)
- 1/4 teaspoon ground black pepper (0.5 g)

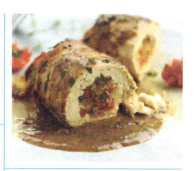

INSTRUCTIONS:

1. Start the oven to 375°F (190°C).
2. In a small skillet, heat half of the olive oil over medium heat. Add the zucchini, red bell pepper, and garlic, and sauté for 3-4 minutes until softened. Remove from heat and let cool slightly.
3. Be cautious not to cut through the chicken breasts when you use a sharp knife to carve a pocket into their sides.
4. Stuff the sautéed vegetable mixture evenly into the pockets of the chicken breasts. Secure with toothpicks if necessary.
5. Brush the chicken breasts with the remaining olive oil and sprinkle with black pepper.
6. In the baking dish, arrange the chicken breasts that have been filled. Bake in an oven that has been warmed for twenty to twenty-five minutes or until the chicken gets an internal temperature of 165 degrees Fahrenheit (74 degrees Celsius).
7. After 5 minutes of resting, take the chicken out of the oven and serve it warm.

Calories: 200
Protein: 31 g
Fat: 7 g
Carbohydrates: 2 g
Sodium: 50 mg
Potassium: 320 mg
Phosphorus: 250 mg

NUTRITIONAL:

TURKEY AND CARROT STEW

 **PREP TIME:** 10 minutes   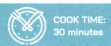 **COOK TIME:** 30 minutes   **SERVINGS:** 2

A hearty and comforting stew with tender turkey, sweet carrots, and fresh parsley.

INGREDIENTS:

- 8 oz turkey breast, cut into bite-sized pieces (225 g)
- 2 medium carrots, sliced (140 g)
- 1 clove garlic, minced (3 g)
- 1 tablespoon olive oil (15 mL)
- 2 cups low-sodium chicken broth (480 mL)
- 1 tablespoon fresh parsley, chopped (4 g)

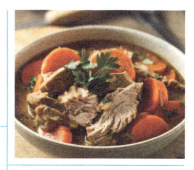

INSTRUCTIONS:

1. Heat the olive oil in a medium-sized pot over medium heat.
2. Brown the turkey chunks on all sides by adding them to the pan and cooking for 5 to 6 minutes while tossing occasionally. Take the turkey out of the oven and place it aside.
3. Chop some garlic and throw some sliced carrots in the same saucepan. Sauté for 2-3 minutes until the garlic is fragrant.
4. Simmer gently after adding the low-sodium chicken broth.
5. Put the browned turkey back in the saucepan, cover it, and simmer the stew for 20-25 minutes, or until the carrots are soft and the turkey is cooked through.
6. Incorporate the chopped parsley and sauté for an additional 1-2 minutes.
7. Remove from heat and serve warm.

Calories: 180
Protein: 28 g
Fat: 5 g
Carbohydrates: 5 g
Sodium: 40 mg
Potassium: 200 mg
Phosphorus: 200 mg

NUTRITIONAL:

LOW SODIUM GRILLED CHICKEN TACOS

 **PREP TIME:** 10 minutes

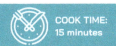 **COOK TIME:** 15 minutes

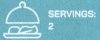 **SERVINGS:** 2

A light and flavorful taco recipe with grilled chicken, fresh lettuce, and a hint of lime, suitable for a renal diet.

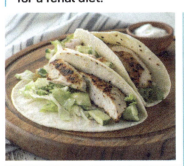

INGREDIENTS:

- 2 boneless, skinless chicken breasts (5 oz / 140 g each)
- 1 tablespoon olive oil (15 mL)
- 1 tablespoon lime juice (15 mL)
- 1/4 teaspoon ground black pepper (0.5 g)
- 2 small white corn tortillas (40 g each)
- 1/2 cup shredded iceberg lettuce (30 g)
- 1/4 cup diced cucumber (40 g)
- 2 tablespoons chopped fresh cilantro (8 g)
- 1 tablespoon sour cream (15 g) (low-phosphorus alternative: plain unsweetened yogurt)

INSTRUCTIONS:

1. Combine lime juice, olive oil, and black pepper in a small bowl.
2. The chicken breasts should be put in a small dish or a resealable plastic bag. Coat them even-ly with the marinade. Let them marinate in the refrigerator for at least 15 minutes.
3. One should heat a grill or grill pan to a temperature of medium-high.
4. Take the chicken out of the marinade and throw away any leftover marinade.
5. Grill the chicken for about 6-7 minutes per side or until it reaches an internal temperature of 165°F (74°C).
6. Let the chicken rest for 5 minutes, then slice it into thin strips.
7. Warm the corn tortillas slightly in a dry pan or on the grill for about 30 seconds per side.
8. Assemble the tacos by placing shredded lettuce, grilled chicken, diced cucumber, and chopped cilantro in each tortilla.
9. Drizzle with a small amount of sour cream or plain yogurt before serving.

NUTRITIONAL:
Calories: 290
Protein: 34 g
Fat: 10 g
Carbohydrates: 18 g
Sodium: 50 mg
Potassium: 320 mg
Phosphorus: 230 mg

CHICKEN WITH ROASTED VEGETABLES

 **PREP TIME:** 10 minutes

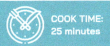 **COOK TIME:** 25 minutes

 SERVINGS: 2

A wholesome dish featuring tender chicken, perfectly roasted zucchini, and red bell pepper.

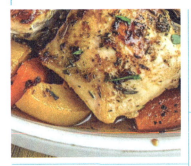

INGREDIENTS:

- 2 boneless, skinless chicken breasts (5 oz / 140 g each)
- 1 medium zucchini, sliced (200 g)
- 1 medium-sized red bell pepper, cut into cubes
- 1 tablespoon olive oil (15 mL)
- 1 clove garlic, minced (3 g)
- 1/4 teaspoon ground black pepper (0.5 g)

INSTRUCTIONS:

1. Start the oven to 400°F (200°C).
2. For the marinade, combine the olive oil, minced garlic, and black pepper in a small bowl.
3. Transfer the chicken breasts, sliced zucchini, and diced red bell pepper to a parchment-lined baking sheet.
4. Drizzle the marinade evenly over the chicken and vegetables, ensuring everything is well coated.
5. After 20 to 25 minutes in a preheated oven, the chicken should be cooked through to an internal temperature of 165 degrees (74 degrees Celsius), and the veggies should be soft and slightly browned.
6. Give the chicken 5 minutes to rest after taking it out of the oven.
7. Serve the chicken alongside the roasted vegetables, garnished with additional parsley if desired.

NUTRITIONAL:
Calories: 210
Protein: 31 g
Fat: 7 g
Carbohydrates: 5 g
Sodium: 60 mg
Potassium: 350 mg
Phosphorus: 250 mg

CHICKEN AND RICE BOWL

 **PREP TIME:** 10 minutes 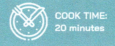 **COOK TIME:** 20 minutes 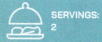 **SERVINGS:** 2

A simple and satisfying meal with tender chicken, fluffy white rice, and light seasoning.

INGREDIENTS:

- 2 boneless, skinless chicken breasts (5 oz / 140 g each)
- 1/2 cup uncooked white rice (85 g)
- 1 tablespoon olive oil (15 mL)
- 1 clove garlic, minced (3 g)
- 1 tablespoon fresh parsley, chopped (4 g)
- 1/4 teaspoon ground black pepper (0.5 g)
- 1 cup water or low-sodium chicken broth (240 mL)

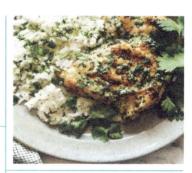

INSTRUCTIONS:

1. In a medium-sized saucepan, bring half of the olive oil to a medium temperature. Add the uncooked white rice and sauté for 1-2 minutes until lightly toasted.
2. Put some water or chicken broth with minimal sodium into the pot. After the water boils, lower the heat to low, cover, and simmer the rice for 15 minutes or until it reaches the desired doneness.
3. In the nonstick pan over medium heat, heat the rest of the olive oil while the rice is cooking. The chicken breasts should be cooked for 6 to 7 minutes on each side or until they hit 165 degrees Fahrenheit (74 degrees Celsius) inside. After taking the chicken out of the pan, let it rest for 5 minutes.
4. Put the minced garlic into the same pan and cook for a minute or until it starts to smell good. Stir in the cooked rice, parsley, and black pepper, mixing well to combine.
5. Before serving, slice the chicken breasts that have rested and top each bowl of rice with them.
6. Warm and top with more parsley, if preferred.

NUTRITIONAL:
Calories: 290
Protein: 32 g
Fat: 7 g
Carbohydrates: 25 g
Sodium: 60 mg
Potassium: 300 mg
Phosphorus: 250 mg

CABBAGE AND CARROT SOUP

 **PREP TIME:** 10 minutes 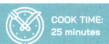 **COOK TIME:** 25 minutes   **SERVINGS:** 4

With the natural sweetness of carrots and the crunch of cabbage, this soup is substantial and comforting.

INGREDIENTS:

- 2 cups chopped cabbage (150 g)
- 1 medium carrot, diced (70 g)
- 1/2 medium onion, finely chopped (50 g)
- 1 clove garlic, minced (3 g)
- 1 tablespoon olive oil (15 mL)
- 4 cups low-sodium vegetable broth (1 L)
- 1/4 teaspoon ground black pepper (0.5 g)

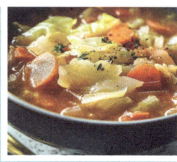

INSTRUCTIONS:

1. Reheat the olive oil in a pot over medium heat.
2. Put the chopped onion and garlic in the pot and sauté for 2 to 3 minutes until the onion is softened and fragrant.
3. Stir in the diced carrot and cook for another 3 minutes, stirring occasionally.
4. Put the chopped cabbage in the pot and mix well with the other vegetables. Cook for 2 minutes to slightly wilt the cabbage.
5. Add the veggie broth with low sodium and bring to a boil over medium heat.
6. Reduce the heat to low, top the pot, and let the soup boil for 15 minutes or until the vegetables are tender.
7. Add the ground black pepper and stir well. Adjust seasoning to taste if necessary.
8. Remove the soup from the heat and serve warm.

NUTRITIONAL:
Calories: 50
Protein: 1 g
Fat: 2 g
Carbohydrates: 7 g
Sodium: 35 mg
Potassium: 120 mg
Phosphorus: 20 mg

GARLIC BASIL CHICKEN SKEWERS

 **PREP TIME:** 12 minutes 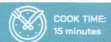 **COOK TIME:** 15 minutes 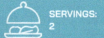 **SERVINGS:** 2

Tender and flavorful chicken skewers marinated with garlic and fresh basil, perfect for grilling or baking.

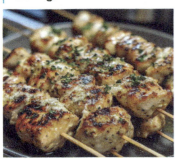

INGREDIENTS:

- half a pound (about 140 grams) of skinless, boneless chicken breasts, diced into bite-sized pieces
- 1 tablespoon olive oil (15 mL)
- 1 clove garlic, minced (3 g)
- 1 tablespoon fresh basil, chopped (4 g)
- 1 teaspoon lemon juice (5 mL)
- 1/4 teaspoon ground black pepper (0.5 g)

INSTRUCTIONS:

1. Marinate the meat in a small basin with olive oil, garlic, basil, lemon juice, and black pepper.
2. Seal the chicken pieces in a plastic bag or arrange them in a shallow dish. Coat the chicken thoroughly by pouring the marinade over it. Marinate in the refrigerator for at least 30 minutes.
3. Heat grill or a grill pan on medium. Put wooden skewers in water for 15 minutes to avoid scorching.
4. Put marinated chicken on skewers.
5. Grill the skewers for 6-7 minutes per side or until the chicken is fully cooked and the internal temperature reaches 165°F (74°C).
6. Rest the skewers for 3-5 minutes after grilling.
7. Serve warm, optionally garnished with additional fresh basil.

NUTRITIONAL:
Calories: 210
Protein: 32 g
Fat: 7 g
Carbohydrates: 1 g
Sodium: 55 mg
Potassium: 300 mg
Phosphorus: 250 mg

CRISPY BAKED CHICKEN NUGGETS

 PREP TIME: 15 minutes 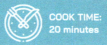 **COOK TIME:** 20 minutes **SERVINGS:** 2

Crunchy and flavorful chicken nuggets baked to perfection for a healthier twist.

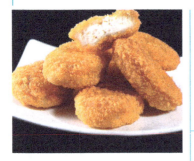

INGREDIENTS:

- 2 boneless, skinless chicken breasts, cut into bite-sized pieces (5 oz / 140 g each)
- 1/4 cup plain breadcrumbs (30 g)
- 1 tablespoon olive oil (15 mL)
- 1/2 teaspoon garlic powder (1 g)
- 1/4 teaspoon ground black pepper (0.5 g)
- 1/4 teaspoon dried parsley (0.5 g)

INSTRUCTIONS:

1. Preheat the oven to 400°F (200°C). Line a baking sheet with parchment paper or lightly grease it with olive oil.
2. In a shallow bowl, mix the breadcrumbs, garlic powder, black pepper, and dried parsley.
3. In another bowl, toss the chicken pieces with olive oil to coat them evenly.
4. Dredge each chicken piece in the breadcrumb mixture, pressing gently to adhere the coating. Place the coated chicken pieces on the prepared baking sheet.
5. Bake in the preheated oven for 18-20 minutes, flipping halfway through, until the chicken nuggets are golden brown and the internal temperature reaches 165°F (74°C).
6. Remove from the oven and let the nuggets cool slightly before serving.

NUTRITIONAL:
Calories: 220
Protein: 30 g
Fat: 6 g
Carbohydrates: 8 g
Sodium: 55 mg
Potassium: 310 mg
Phosphorus: 240 mg

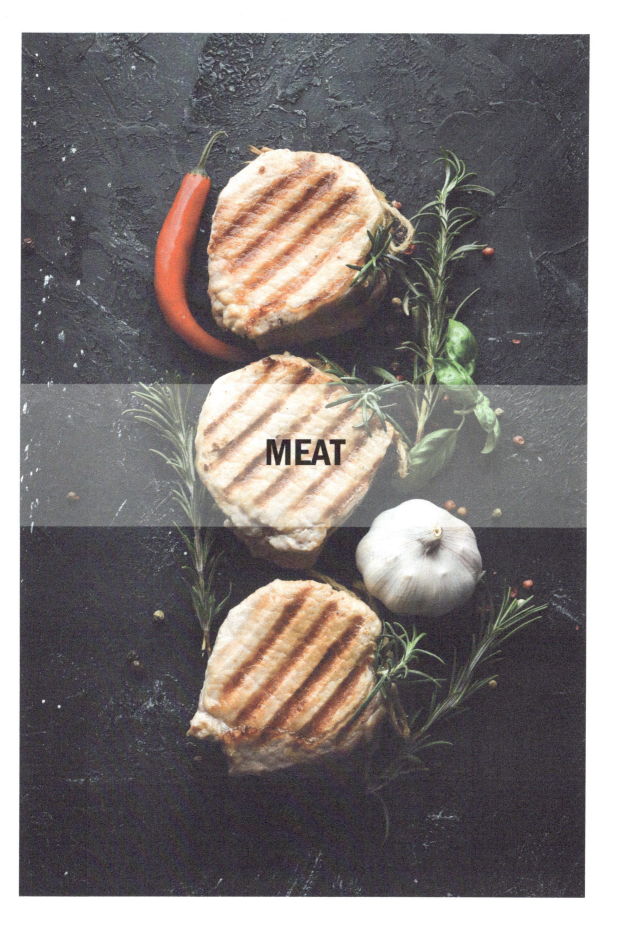

MEAT

GARLIC HERB BEEF STIR-FRY

 **PREP TIME:** 10 minutes    **COOK TIME:** 15 minutes   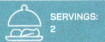 **SERVINGS:** 2

A savory and quick stir-fry with tender beef, fresh zucchini, and aromatic herbs.

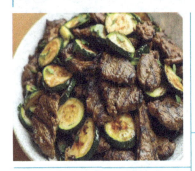

INGREDIENTS:

- 8 oz lean beef, cut into thin strips (225 g)
- 1 medium zucchini, sliced into half-moons (200 g)
- 1 tablespoon olive oil (15 mL)
- 1 clove garlic, minced (3 g)
- 1 tablespoon fresh parsley, chopped (4 g)
- 1/4 teaspoon ground black pepper (0.5 g)

INSTRUCTIONS:

1. In a large-sized skillet, heat half of the olive oil over medium-high heat.
2. Put the beef strips in the skillet and stir-fry for 4-5 minutes or until browned and cooked to your desired doneness. After taking the steak out of the skillet, place it aside.
3. In this skillet, add the remaining olive oil and the minced garlic. Sauté for 1 minute until fragrant.
4. Stir-fry the zucchini in the skillet for three to four minutes or until it is soft but still has a tiny crunch.
5. Return the beef to the skillet and sprinkle with fresh parsley and black pepper. Stir well to combine.
6. Cook for an extra 1-2 minutes to heat through.
7. Remove from heat and serve immediately.

NUTRITIONAL:
Calories: 230
Protein: 27 g
Fat: 10 g
Carbohydrates: 3 g
Sodium: 50 mg
Potassium: 350 mg
Phosphorus: 220 mg

BALSAMIC GLAZED PORK TENDERLOIN

 **PREP TIME:** 10 minutes   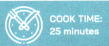 **COOK TIME:** 25 minutes   **SERVINGS:** 2

A tender and flavorful pork dish with a rich balsamic glaze infused with garlic and thyme.

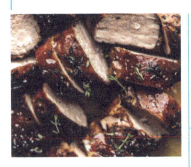

INGREDIENTS:

- 1 pork tenderloin (10 oz / 280 g)
- 2 tablespoons balsamic vinegar (30 mL)
- 1 tablespoon olive oil (15 mL)
- 1 clove garlic, minced (3 g)
- 1/2 teaspoon dried thyme (1 g)
- 1/4 teaspoon ground black pepper (0.5 g)

INSTRUCTIONS:

1. Reheat the oven to 375°F (or 190°C).
2. In a small-sized bowl, mix the balsamic vinegar, olive oil, minced garlic, dried thyme, and black pepper to create the glaze.
3. Heat an oven-safe skillet over medium-high heat. Add a small amount of olive oil if needed. Sear the pork tenderloin for 2-3 minutes on each side until golden brown.
4. Brush the balsamic glaze evenly over the pork tenderloin.
5. After the oven has been warmed, place the pan inside and roast the pig for 25 minutes or until its internal temp reaches 145°F (63°C).
6. Before slicing, take the pan out of the oven and give the pork five minutes to rest.
7. Serve warm, optionally garnished with additional thyme or a drizzle of the pan juices.

NUTRITIONAL:
Calories: 200
Protein: 30 g
Fat: 7 g
Carbohydrates: 2 g
Sodium: 50 mg
Potassium: 350 mg
Phosphorus: 250 mg

ROSEMARY GARLIC LAMB CHOPS

 **PREP TIME:** 10 minutes   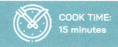 **COOK TIME:** 15 minutes   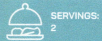 **SERVINGS:** 2

Aromatic and tender lamb chops infused with the rich flavors of garlic and rosemary.

INGREDIENTS:

- 4 lamb chops (5 oz / 140 g each)
- 1 tablespoon olive oil (15 mL)
- 2 cloves garlic, minced (6 g)
- 1 teaspoon fresh rosemary, chopped (2 g)
- 1/4 teaspoon ground black pepper (0.5 g)

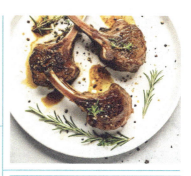

INSTRUCTIONS:

1. In a small-sized bowl, mix the olive oil, minced garlic, chopped rosemary, and ground black pepper to create a marinade.
2. Rub the marinade evenly over the lamb chops, ensuring all sides are coated. The lamb chops should marinate in the fridge for at least 15 minutes while covered.
3. Reheat a skillet or grill pan on medium-high heat.
4. To get medium-rare, place the lamb chops in the skillet and cook for 4 minutes on each side or until they are done to your liking. Make sure the internal temp reaches 145°F (63°C) for medium by using a meat thermometer.
5. Remove the lamb chops from the skillet and let them rest for 5 minutes before serving.
6. Serve warm, optionally garnished with additional rosemary sprigs.

Calories: 300
Protein: 28 g
Fat: 20 g
Carbohydrates: 1 g
Sodium: 70 mg
Potassium: 250 mg
Phosphorus: 220 mg

NUTRITIONAL:

BEEF AND CAULIFLOWER RICE BOWL

 PREP TIME: 10 minutes   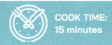 **COOK TIME:** 15 minutes    **SERVINGS:** 2

A quick and nutritious dish combining savory ground beef with tender cauliflower rice and fresh parsley.

INGREDIENTS:

- 8 oz ground beef (225 g, lean)
- 2 cups riced cauliflower (200 g)
- 1 tablespoon olive oil (15 mL)
- 1 clove garlic, minced (3 g)
- 1 tablespoon fresh parsley, chopped (4 g)

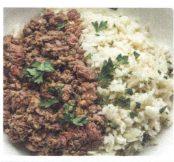

INSTRUCTIONS:

1. In a large-sized skillet, heat half of the olive oil over medium heat.
2. Put the ground beef and cook for 8 minutes, breaking it up with a spatula, until browned and fully cooked. After taking the steak out of the skillet, place it aside.
3. In this skillet, add the remaining olive oil and minced garlic. Sauté for 1 minute until fragrant.
4. Cook, stirring occasionally, until the riced cauliflower is soft and lightly browned, for 7 minutes.
5. Put the cauliflower rice in the skillet along with the cooked meat beef. To blend the flavors, add the chopped parsley and simmer for one to two more minutes.
6. Serve warm, optionally garnished with additional parsley.

Calories: 220
Protein: 22 g
Fat: 12 g
Carbohydrates: 5 g
Sodium: 50 mg
Potassium: 250 mg
Phosphorus: 200 mg

NUTRITIONAL:

LEMON PEPPER PORK CHOPS

 **PREP TIME:** 10 minutes   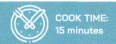 **COOK TIME:** 15 minutes   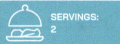 **SERVINGS:** 2

A zesty and flavorful dish with juicy pork chops infused with lemon and black pepper.

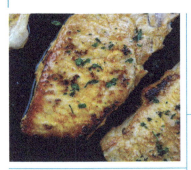

INGREDIENTS:

- 2 pork chops (6 oz / 170 g each, bone-in or boneless)
- 1 tablespoon olive oil (15 mL)
- 1 tablespoon lemon juice (15 mL)
- 1/4 teaspoon ground black pepper (0.5 g)
- 1 tablespoon fresh parsley, chopped (4 g)

INSTRUCTIONS:

1. In a small-sized bowl, whisk together the olive oil, lemon juice, and some black pepper to make the marinade.
2. Put the cuts of pork in a plastic bag that can be closed or on a shallow plate. Make sure they are uniformly covered after pouring the marinade over them. Give the pork chops at least fifteen minutes to marinate in the fridge.
3. Reheat a skillet or grill pan on medium-high heat.
4. After taking the pork chops out of the marinade, let any extra drip off. Throw away any remaining marinade.
5. Cook the pork chops for 6-7 minutes per side or until they reach an internal temp of 145°F (63°C) for medium doneness.
6. After taking the pork chops off of the stove, give them five minutes to rest.
7. Garnish with fresh parsley and serve warm.

NUTRITIONAL:
Calories: 260
Protein: 28 g
Fat: 14 g
Carbohydrates: 1 g
Sodium: 55 mg
Potassium: 330 mg
Phosphorus: 250 mg

HERBED MEATBALLS

 **PREP TIME:** 10 minutes   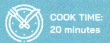 **COOK TIME:** 20 minutes   **SERVINGS:** 2

Flavorful and tender meatballs infused with fresh parsley and garlic, perfect for a hearty meal.

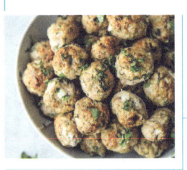

INGREDIENTS:

- 8 oz ground beef or pork (225 g, lean)
- 1 small egg (1.75 oz / 50 g)
- 2 tablespoons breadcrumbs (15 g, limited)
- 1 tablespoon fresh parsley, chopped (4 g)
- 1/2 teaspoon garlic powder (1 g)

INSTRUCTIONS:

1. Reheat the oven to 375°F (or 190°C) and line a baking pan with one sheet of parchment paper.
2. In a bowl, mix the ground beef or pork, egg, breadcrumbs, parsley, and garlic powder. Mix until all ingredients are evenly incorporated. Avoid overmixing.
3. Form the mixture into small meatballs, about 2.5 cm in diameter, and put them on the prepared baking sheet.
4. For 18 to 20 minutes or until the meatballs are cooked through and have an internal temp of 160°F (71°C), bake them in a preheated oven.
5. Remove from the oven and let the meatballs cool for a few minutes before serving.
6. Serve warm, optionally garnished with additional parsley or paired with a kidney-friendly sauce or side dish.

NUTRITIONAL:
Calories: 220
Protein: 20 g
Fat: 12 g
Carbohydrates: 4 g
Sodium: 50 mg
Potassium: 200 mg
Phosphorus: 180 mg

BEEF AND ZUCCHINI SKILLET

 **PREP TIME:** 10 minutes    **COOK TIME:** 15 minutes   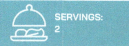 **SERVINGS:** 2

A quick and hearty dish with savory ground beef and tender zucchini, enhanced with garlic and thyme.

INGREDIENTS:

- 8 oz ground beef (225 g, lean)
- 1 medium zucchini, sliced into half-moons (200 g)
- 1 tablespoon olive oil (15 mL)
- 1 clove garlic, minced (3 g)
- 1/2 teaspoon dried thyme (1 g)
- 1/4 teaspoon ground black pepper (0.5 g)

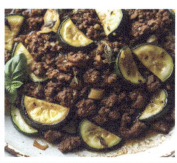

INSTRUCTIONS:

1. In a large-sized skillet, heat half of the olive oil over medium heat.
2. Put the ground beef in the skillet and cook for 6-7 minutes, breaking it up with a spatula, until browned and fully cooked. After taking the steak out of the skillet, place it aside.
3. In this skillet, add the remaining olive oil and minced garlic. Sauté for 1 minute until fragrant.
4. Add the zucchini slices and sprinkle with dried thyme and black pepper. Cook, stirring periodically, until the zucchini is soft but still has a tiny crunch after 5 minutes.
5. After cooking, add the ground beef back to the skillet and mix it with the zucchini. To ensure it is well heated, cook for a further one to two minutes.
6. Remove from heat and serve warm.

Calories: 220
Protein: 22 g
Fat: 12 g
Carbohydrates: 3 g
Sodium: 40 mg
Potassium: 250 mg
Phosphorus: 200 mg

NUTRITIONAL:

BEEF STEW WITH CARROTS AND MUSHROOMS

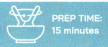 **PREP TIME:** 15 minutes   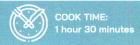 **COOK TIME:** 1 hour 30 minutes   **SERVINGS:** 2

A hearty and comforting stew with tender beef, sweet carrots, and earthy mushrooms.

INGREDIENTS:

- 8 oz lean beef stew meat, cubed (225 g)
- 1 medium carrot, sliced (70 g)
- 1/2 cup sliced mushrooms (50 g)
- 1 tablespoon olive oil (15 mL)
- 1 clove garlic, minced (3 g)
- 2 cups low-sodium beef broth (480 mL)
- 1/4 teaspoon dried thyme (0.5 g)
- 1/4 teaspoon ground black pepper (0.5 g)

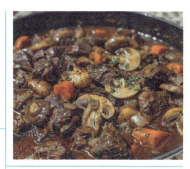

INSTRUCTIONS:

1. Preheat 1 tablespoon olive oil (15 mL) in a large pot on medium-high heat.
2. After adding the meat cubes to the saucepan, cook them for five to seven minutes, browning on both sides. Set aside the meat after removing it.
3. In this pot, add the minced garlic and sauté for 1 minute until fragrant.
4. Put the carrots and mushrooms in the pot, cooking for 3-4 minutes while stirring occasionally.
5. Add the low-sodium beef broth to the saucepan with the browned meat.
6. Sprinkle in the dried thyme and black pepper, stirring to combine.
7. When bringing the mixture to a boil, reduce the heat. For one hour, cover and simmer, stirring periodically, until the veggies are cooked through and the meat is soft.
8. Serve warm, adjusting spice to taste.

Calories: 220
Protein: 25 g
Fat: 9 g
Carbohydrates: 5 g
Sodium: 60 mg
Potassium: 300 mg
Phosphorus: 200 mg

NUTRITIONAL:

SLOW-COOKED PULLED PORK

 **PREP TIME:** 10 minutes

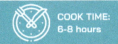 **COOK TIME:** 6-8 hours

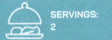 **SERVINGS:** 2

A tender and flavorful pulled pork dish infused with garlic and apple cider vinegar, perfect for a slow cooker.

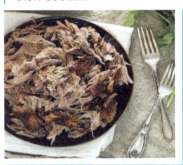

INGREDIENTS:

- 12 oz pork shoulder (340 g)
- 1 tablespoon apple cider vinegar (15 mL)
- 1 clove garlic, minced (3 g)
- 1/2 teaspoon onion powder (1 g)
- 1/4 teaspoon ground black pepper (0.5 g)

INSTRUCTIONS:

1. With a piece of paper towel, pat dry the pork shoulder. Rub the minced garlic, onion powder, and black pepper evenly over the pork.
2. Place the shoulder of the pork in a slow cooker. Drizzle the apple cider vinegar over the pork.
3. Add 1/4 cup (60 mL) of water to the slow cooker to prevent sticking.
4. Cover and cook on low for 6-8 hours or until the pork is tender and easily pulls apart with a fork.
5. When done, take the pork out of the slow cooker and use two forks to shred it.
6. Put the pork shreds back in the slow cooker and stir them with the cooking liquids to keep them moist.
7. Serve warm, either on its own or as a filling for a kidney-friendly wrap or alongside roasted vegetables.

NUTRITIONAL:
Calories: 300
Protein: 30 g
Fat: 20 g
Carbohydrates: 1 g
Sodium: 60 mg
Potassium: 350 mg
Phosphorus: 220 mg

GREEK LAMB WITH ORZO

 **PREP TIME:** 15 minutes

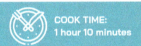 **COOK TIME:** 1 hour 10 minutes

 SERVINGS: 2

A flavorful Greek-inspired dish featuring tender lamb and orzo seasoned with herbs and garlic.

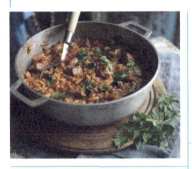

INGREDIENTS:

- 8 oz lamb shoulder or leg, cut into cubes (225 g)
- 1/2 cup uncooked orzo (85 g)
- 1 tablespoon olive oil (15 mL)
- 1 clove garlic, minced (3 g)
- 1/4 teaspoon dried oregano (0.5 g)
- 1/4 teaspoon ground black pepper (0.5 g)
- 2 cups low-sodium chicken broth (480 mL)
- 1 tablespoon fresh parsley, chopped (4 g)

INSTRUCTIONS:

1. In a Dutch oven or pan, reheat the olive oil over medium heat.
2. Put the lamb cubes in the skillet and brown them on all sides for about 6-8 minutes. Remove the lamb and set aside.
3. In this skillet, add the minced garlic and sauté for 1 minute until fragrant.
4. Put the lamb back in the skillet and season with black pepper and dried oregano. Stir to properly distribute the spices over the lamb.
5. Bring the mixture to a boil after adding the low-sodium chicken broth. The lamb should be tender after 45 to 50 minutes of simmering on low heat with a lid on.
6. Add the orzo and simmer, uncovered, stirring occasionally, for 10 to 12 minutes or until the orzo is soft and the broth has mostly been absorbed.
7. Before serving, take off the heat and sprinkle some fresh parsley on top.

NUTRITIONAL:
Calories: 320
Protein: 25 g
Fat: 12 g
Carbohydrates: 28 g
Sodium: 55 mg
Potassium: 280 mg
Phosphorus: 210 mg

LAMB KEBAB WITH SAUCE

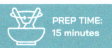 **PREP TIME:** 15 minutes

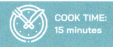 **COOK TIME:** 15 minutes

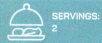 **SERVINGS:** 2

Succulent lamb kebabs served with a tangy and herbaceous sauce, perfect for grilling or baking.

INGREDIENTS:

For the Lamb Kebab:
- 8 oz lamb, cut into bite-sized pieces (225 g)
- 1 tablespoon olive oil (15 mL)
- 1 clove garlic, minced (3 g)
- 1 teaspoon fresh rosemary, chopped (2 g)
- 1/4 teaspoon ground black pepper (0.5 g)

For the Sauce:
- 2 tablespoons plain unsweetened yogurt (30 mL)
- 1 teaspoon lemon juice (5 mL)
- 1 tablespoon fresh parsley, chopped (4 g)
- 1/4 teaspoon garlic powder (0.5 g)

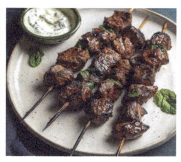

INSTRUCTIONS:

For the Lamb Kebab:
1. In a small-sized bowl, whisk together the olive oil, minced garlic, chopped rosemary, and black pepper to make the marinade.
2. Put the lamb pieces in the marinade, ensuring all pieces are coated. Cover and refrigerate for at least 30 minutes.
3. Preheat a grill or grill pan to medium heat. To avoid scorching, immerse wooden skewers in water for fifteen minutes.
4. Thread the marinated lamb pieces onto skewers.
5. The lamb should be cooked to your preferred doneness (medium-rare: 145°F / 63°C, medium: 160°F / 71°C) after 6 to 8 minutes of grilling, flipping periodically.
6. Before serving, take the kebabs from the grill and let them rest for five minutes.

For the Sauce:
7. In a small-sized bowl, mix the yogurt, lemon juice, chopped parsley, and garlic powder until well combined.
8. Serve the sauce on the side or drizzle over the kebabs.

NUTRITIONAL:
Calories: 290
Protein: 26 g
Fat: 16 g
Carbohydrates: 3 g
Sodium: 60 mg
Potassium: 250 mg
Phosphorus: 220 mg

GINGER SPICED LAMB CHOPS

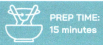 **PREP TIME:** 15 minutes

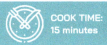 **COOK TIME:** 15 minutes

 SERVINGS: 2

Tender and flavorful lamb chops marinated with aromatic ginger and warm spices.

INGREDIENTS:

- 4 lamb chops (5 oz / 140 g each)
- 1 tablespoon olive oil (15 mL)
- 1 teaspoon fresh ginger, grated (5 g)
- 1/2 teaspoon ground cinnamon (1 g)
- 1/4 teaspoon ground cumin (0.5 g)
- 1/4 teaspoon ground black pepper (0.5 g)

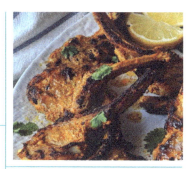

INSTRUCTIONS:

1. In a small-sized bowl, mix the olive oil, grated ginger, ground cinnamon, ground cumin, and black pepper to create a marinade.
2. Evenly coat the lamb chops on every side with the marinade. To allow the flavors to combine, cover and chill for at least half an hour.
3. Reheat a skillet or grill pan over medium-high heat.
4. Cook the lamb chops for 4-5 minutes each side or until they reach your desired level of doneness (medium-rare: 145°F / 63°C, medium: 160°F / 71°C).
5. Replace the lamb chops from the pan and allow them to rest for 4 minutes before serving.
6. Serve warm, optionally garnished with fresh parsley or a wedge of lemon for added brightness.

NUTRITIONAL:
Calories: 310
Protein: 27 g
Fat: 21 g
Carbohydrates: 1 g
Sodium: 50 mg
Potassium: 240 mg
Phosphorus: 210 mg

MEDITERRANEAN LAMB PATTIES

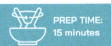 PREP TIME:
15 minutes

 COOK TIME:
10 minutes

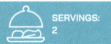 SERVINGS:
2

Mediterranean-flavored, succulent lamb patties that are ideal for a quick and filling supper.

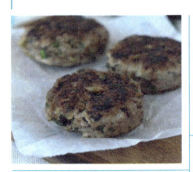

INGREDIENTS:

- 8 oz ground lamb (225 g)
- 1 tablespoon fresh parsley, chopped (4 g)
- 1 teaspoon dried oregano (1 g)
- 1 clove garlic, minced (3 g)
- 1/4 teaspoon ground black pepper (0.5 g)
- 1/2 teaspoon lemon zest (1 g)
- 1 teaspoon olive oil (5 mL)

INSTRUCTIONS:

1. In a large bowl, combine parsley, ground lamb, oregano, minced garlic, black pepper, and lemon zest. Mix until all components are evenly distributed.
2. Separate the mixture into four parts, and then shape each into a patty that is about 1/2 inch (1.25 cm) thick.
3. Reheat the olive oil in a non-stick skillet on medium heat.
4. Add the lamb patties to the skillet and cook for 4-5 minutes on each side or until browned and cooked through to your desired doneness (medium: 160°F / 71°C).
5. Replace the patties from the skillet and allow them to rest for 4 minutes before serving.
6. Serve warm, optionally garnished with additional parsley or paired with a side of roasted vegetables or a light salad.

NUTRITIONAL:
Calories: 280
Protein: 22 g
Fat: 21 g
Carbohydrates: 1 g
Sodium: 50 mg
Potassium: 200 mg
Phosphorus: 180 mg

STUFFED BELL PEPPERS WITH BEEF

 PREP TIME:
15 minutes

 COOK TIME:
30 minutes

SERVINGS:
2

A hearty and wholesome dish featuring bell peppers filled with a flavorful mixture of beef, rice, and vegetables.

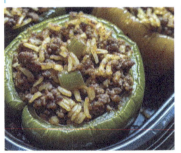

INGREDIENTS:

- 2 large red bell peppers (200 g each)
- 8 oz ground beef (225 g, lean)
- 1/2 cup cooked brown rice (85 g)
- 1/4 cup finely diced carrot (40 g)
- 1/4 cup finely chopped onion (40 g)
- 1 clove garlic, minced (3 g)
- 1 tablespoon olive oil (15 mL)
- 1 tablespoon fresh parsley, chopped (4 g)

INSTRUCTIONS:

1. Reheat the oven to 375°F (or 190°C).
2. Slice off the red bell peppers' tops, and then take out the seeds and membranes. Place the peppers on the side.
3. Reheat the olive oil in a large pan on medium-high heat. Add the onion, carrot, and garlic, and sauté for 3-4 minutes until softened.
4. Put the ground beef in the skillet and cook for 5-7 minutes, breaking it up with a spatula, until browned and cooked through.
5. Stir in the cooked brown rice and parsley, mixing well to combine. Remove the skillet from heat.
6. Stuff the beef and rice mixture evenly into the prepared bell peppers.
7. Put the stuffed peppers upright in a baking dish. Pour water (about 1/4 cup) into the bottom of the dish to keep the peppers moist.
8. Bake the dish for 25 minutes in a preheated oven after covering it with foil. To gently brown the tops, take off the foil and continue baking for another five minutes.
9. Before serving, take the peppers out of the oven and allow them to cool somewhat.

NUTRITIONAL:
Calories: 280
Protein: 22 g
Fat: 12 g
Carbohydrates: 20 g
Sodium: 50 mg
Potassium: 350 mg
Phosphorus: 200 mg

KIDNEY-FRIENDLY BEEF BOURGUIGNON

 **PREP TIME:** 15 minutes   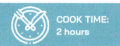 **COOK TIME:** 2 hours   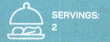 **SERVINGS:** 2

A modified version of the traditional French meal with rich tastes and delicate meat that is suited for a kidney-friendly diet.

INGREDIENTS:

- 8 oz lean beef stew meat, cubed (225 g)
- 1 tablespoon olive oil (15 mL)
- 1/2 cup pearl onions, peeled (70 g)
- 1/2 cup sliced mushrooms (50 g)
- 1 medium carrot, sliced (70 g)
- 1 clove garlic, minced (3 g)
- 1 tablespoon all-purpose flour (8 g)
- 1/2 cup low-sodium beef broth (120 mL)
- 1/2 cup water (120 mL)
- 1 teaspoon dried thyme (1 g)
- 1/4 teaspoon ground black pepper (0.5 g)

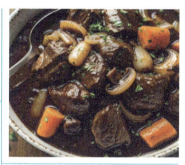

INSTRUCTIONS:

1. Reheat 1 tablespoon olive oil (15 mL) in a pot or Dutch oven on medium-high heat.
2. After adding the meat cubes, cook for 5 to 7 minutes, browning them on both sides. After taking the steak out of the saucepan, set it aside.
3. In this pot, add the pearl onions, mushrooms, and carrots. Sauté for 3-4 minutes until slightly softened.
4. Add the minced garlic and sauté until it becomes fragrant, about 1 minute.
5. To coat the veggies, sprinkle them with flour and give them a good swirl. Cook for one minute to eliminate the flavor of uncooked flour.
6. Gradually add the low-sodium beef broth and water, stirring constantly to prevent lumps.
7. Return the browned beef to the pot. Add the dried thyme and black pepper, stirring to combine.
8. Reduce the heat to low after bringing the mixture to a mild boil. Simmer, covered, stirring periodically, until the meat is cooked and the sauce is thickened, about 1 to 2 hours.
9. Adjust seasoning if needed, and serve warm with a side of kidney-friendly bread or a light vegetable dish.

Calories: 260
Protein: 25 g
Fat: 11 g
Carbohydrates: 7 g
Sodium: 55 mg
Potassium: 240 mg
Phosphorus: 200 mg

NUTRITIONAL:

SMOTHERED PORK CHOPS AND SAUTÉED GREENS

 **PREP TIME:** 15 minutes   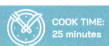 **COOK TIME:** 25 minutes   **SERVINGS:** 2

A comforting dish of tender pork chops smothered in a flavorful sauce served with lightly sautéed greens.

INGREDIENTS:

- For the Pork Chops:
- 2 boneless pork chops (6 oz / 170 g each)
- 1 tablespoon olive oil (15 mL)
- 1/4 cup of low-sodium chicken broth (60 mL)
- 1/4 cup of unsweetened almond milk (60 mL)
- 1/2 teaspoon garlic powder (1 g)
- 1/4 teaspoon onion powder (0.5 g)
- 1/4 teaspoon ground black pepper (0.5 g)
- For the Sautéed Greens:
- 2 cups chopped collard greens or kale (200 g)
- 1 teaspoon olive oil (5 mL)
- 1 clove garlic, minced (3 g)
- 1/8 teaspoon ground black pepper (0.25 g)

INSTRUCTIONS:

For the Pork Chops:
1. Reheat the olive oil in a skillet over medium heat.
2. Garnish the pork chops with garlic powder, onion powder, and black pepper.
3. Set the pork chops in the skillet and sear them until golden brown, 3–4 minutes per side. Replace the pork chops from the skillet and set aside.
4. In the same skillet, reduce the heat to low and add the low-sodium chicken broth and almond milk. Bring the sauce to a slow simmer after stirring it.
5. Place the pork chops back in the skillet, cover, and simmer until they are soft and cooked through about 8 to 10 minutes.

For the Sautéed Greens:
6. Reheat the olive oil in a separate skillet over medium heat.
7. Add the minced garlic and sauté for 1 minute until fragrant.
8. Add the chopped greens and cook for 5-7 minutes, stirring occasionally, until wilted and tender. Sprinkle with black pepper and stir to combine.

To Serve:
9. Plate the smothered pork chops with the sautéed greens on the side.
10. Drizzle some of the sauce over the pork chops and enjoy warm.

Calories: 260
Protein: 30 g
Fat: 10 g
Carbohydrates: 5 g
Sodium: 55 mg
Potassium: 300 mg
Phosphorus: 230 mg

NUTRITIONAL:

CRANBERRY SPARE RIBS (PORK)

 **PREP TIME:** 15 minutes   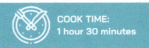 **COOK TIME:** 1 hour 30 minutes   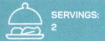 **SERVINGS:** 2

A sweet and tangy dish with tender pork spare ribs coated in a flavorful cranberry glaze.

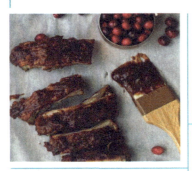

INGREDIENTS:

- 12 oz pork spare ribs, trimmed (340 g)
- 1/4 cup unsweetened cranberry juice (60 mL)
- 2 tablespoons honey or a kidney-friendly sweetener (30 mL)
- 1 clove garlic, minced (3 g)
- 1/2 teaspoon ground black pepper (0.5 g)
- 1/4 teaspoon ground cinnamon (0.5 g)

INSTRUCTIONS:

1. Prepare the Spare Ribs: eheat the oven to 350°F (175°C). Line a baking dish with foil.
2. Season the pork spare ribs with ground black pepper and place them in the baking dish. Bake the dish for one hour after covering it with foil.
3. Make the Cranberry Glaze: Add the honey, ground cinnamon, minced garlic, and unsweetened cranberry juice to a small saucepan set over medium heat. Simmer until the sauce thickens slightly, stirring regularly, for 7 minutes. Take off the heat.
4. Glaze the Ribs: After an hour of baking, take off the foil and liberally coat the ribs with the cranberry glaze. Uncover the ribs and bake them for another 20 to 30 minutes, basting them with glaze every 10 minutes.
5. Serve: Before serving, take the ribs out of the oven and let them rest for five minutes. Garnish with additional glaze if desired.

NUTRITIONAL:
Calories: 300
Protein: 25 g
Fat: 18 g
Carbohydrates: 10 g
Sodium: 60 mg
Potassium: 250 mg
Phosphorus: 200 mg

STEWED PORK CHOPS WITH APPLES AND CINNAMON

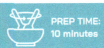 **PREP TIME:** 10 minutes   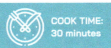 **COOK TIME:** 30 minutes   **SERVINGS:** 2

Tender pork chops simmered with sweet apples and warm cinnamon for a comforting and flavorful dish.

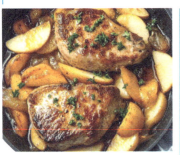

INGREDIENTS:

- 2 boneless pork chops (6 oz / 170 g each)
- 1 medium apple, peeled and thinly sliced (150 g)
- 1/2 teaspoon ground cinnamon (1 g)
- 1 tablespoon olive oil (15 mL)
- 1 clove garlic, minced (3 g)
- 1/4 cup of low-sodium chicken broth (60 mL)
- 1 teaspoon honey or kidney-friendly sweetener (5 mL, optional)

INSTRUCTIONS:

1. Reheat 1 tablespoon olive oil (15 mL) in a large skillet over medium heat.
2. Season the pork chops with ground black pepper if desired, and sear them in the skillet for 2-3 minutes per side until golden brown. Remove the pork chops and set aside.
3. In this skillet, add the minced garlic and sauté for 1 minute until fragrant.
4. Add the sliced apples and sprinkle with ground cinnamon. Cook for 5 minutes, stirring periodically, until the apples begin to soften.
5. Stir in the low-sodium chicken broth and honey (if using). Bring the mixture to a gentle simmer.
6. Put the pork chops back in the skillet with the apples nestled in between them. The pork chops should be cooked and tender after 15 to 20 minutes of simmering over low heat with a lid on (internal temperature should reach 145°F/63°C).
7. Take off the heat and give the dish five minutes to rest.
8. Serve warm, spooning the apple-cinnamon sauce over the pork chops.

NUTRITIONAL:
Calories: 250
Protein: 28 g
Fat: 12 g
Carbohydrates: 6 g
Sodium: 55 mg
Potassium: 260 mg
Phosphorus: 200 mg

BEEF AND ZUCCHINI MEATLOAF

 **PREP TIME:** 15 minutes   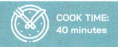 **COOK TIME:** 40 minutes   **SERVINGS:** 2

A moist and flavorful meatloaf with added zucchini for a healthy twist.

INGREDIENTS:

- 8 oz ground beef (225 g, lean)
- 1/2 cup grated zucchini (75 g)
- 1 small egg (50 g)
- 2 tablespoons breadcrumbs (15 g, limited)
- 1 tablespoon fresh parsley, chopped (4 g)
- 1/4 teaspoon ground black pepper (0.5 g)

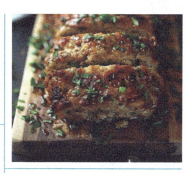

INSTRUCTIONS:

1. Reheat an oven to 375°F (190°C). Lightly grease a small loaf pan or line it with parchment paper.
2. In a large-sized mixing bowl, combine the ground beef, grated zucchini, egg, breadcrumbs, parsley, and black pepper. Mix until all ingredients are evenly incorporated.
3. Replace the mixture with the prepared loaf pan, pressing it down lightly to form a uniform shape.
4. The meatloaf should be baked for 40 minutes in a preheated oven or until it is well cooked and the internal temperature reaches 160°F (71°C).
5. Replace the meatloaf from the oven and let it rest for 5 minutes before slicing.
6. Serve warm, optionally garnished with additional parsley.

Calories: 220
Protein: 25 g
Fat: 10 g
Carbohydrates: 5 g
Sodium: 50 mg
Potassium: 200 mg
Phosphorus: 180 mg

NUTRITIONAL:

ONION SMOTHERED STEAK

 **PREP TIME:** 10 minutes   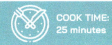 **COOK TIME:** 25 minutes   **SERVINGS:** 2

A tender and juicy steak topped with caramelized onions for a rich and savory flavor.

INGREDIENTS:

- 8 oz beef steak (225 g, such as sirloin or round)
- 1 medium onion, thinly sliced (100 g)
- 1 tablespoon olive oil (15 mL)
- 1/4 teaspoon garlic powder (0.5 g)
- 1/4 teaspoon ground black pepper (0.5 g)
- 1/4 cup low-sodium beef broth (60 mL)

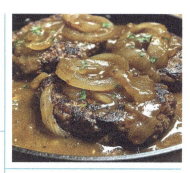

INSTRUCTIONS:

1. Reheat half of the olive oil in a skillet over medium heat.
2. Season the steak with garlic powder and black pepper on both sides.
3. Sear the steak in the skillet for 3-4 minutes per side or until it reaches your desired doneness (medium-rare: 145°F / 63°C, medium: 160°F / 71°C). Replace the steak from the skillet and let it rest.
4. In this skillet, add the remaining olive oil and sliced onions. Cook over medium heat, stirring periodically, for 10 minutes or until the onions are soft and golden brown.
5. Stir the skillet after adding the low-sodium beef broth, making sure to scrape off any browned pieces from the pan's bottom. Simmer for 2-3 minutes until slightly thickened.
6. Return the steak to the skillet and spoon the onion mixture over it. Cook for an extra 2 minutes to heat through.
7. Serve the steak topped with the smothered onions.

Calories: 250
Protein: 28 g
Fat: 12 g
Carbohydrates: 4 g
Sodium: 50 mg
Potassium: 300 mg
Phosphorus: 220 mg

NUTRITIONAL:

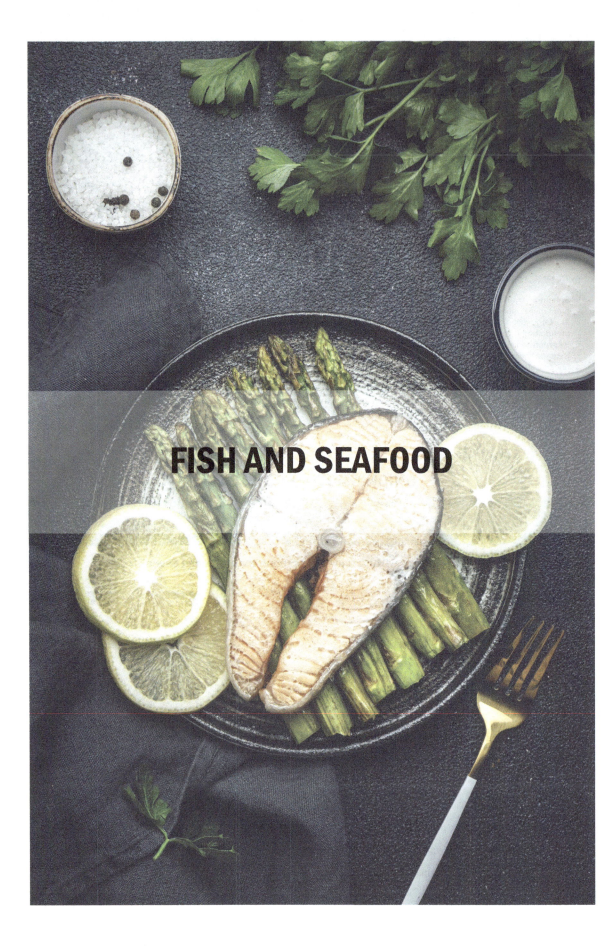

FISH AND SEAFOOD

LINGUINE WITH GARLIC AND SHRIMP

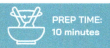 **PREP TIME:** 10 minutes   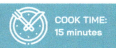 **COOK TIME:** 15 minutes   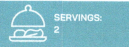 **SERVINGS:** 2

A simple yet elegant pasta dish with tender shrimp and a flavorful garlic-infused sauce.

INGREDIENTS:

- 4 oz linguine (115 g, dry)
- 6 oz shrimp, peeled and deveined (170 g)
- 2 tablespoons olive oil (30 mL)
- 2 cloves garlic, minced (6 g)
- 1/4 teaspoon ground black pepper (0.5 g)
- 1 tablespoon fresh parsley, chopped (4 g)
- 1/4 teaspoon with red pepper flakes (optional for heat)

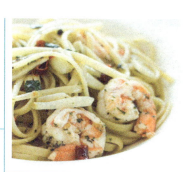

INSTRUCTIONS:

1. As directed on the package, bring a big pot of water to a boil and cook the linguine until it's al dente. Drain and set aside, reserving 1/4 cup of the pasta water.
2. Reheat 1 tablespoon of olive oil in a large skillet over medium heat. Put the shrimp and cook for 3 minutes per side or until pink and opaque. Transfer the shrimp from the skillet and set aside.
3. In this skillet, add the remaining olive oil and minced garlic. Sauté for 1-2 minutes until fragrant, being careful not to burn the garlic. To make a light sauce, add the pasta water that was set aside to the skillet.
4. Coat the cooked shrimp with the garlic sauce by returning them to the skillet and stirring. Gently throw the drained linguine into the pan to mix it up.
5. Sprinkle with ground black pepper, fresh parsley, and red pepper flakes (if using). Toss again to ensure the flavors are evenly distributed.
6. Divide the linguine and shrimp between two plates and serve warm.

NUTRITIONAL:
Calories: 320
Protein: 24 g
Fat: 10 g
Carbohydrates: 36 g
Sodium: 150 mg
Potassium: 200 mg
Phosphorus: 190 mg

BROILED MAPLE SALMON FILLET

 **PREP TIME:** 10 minutes   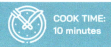 **COOK TIME:** 10 minutes   **SERVINGS:** 2

A sweet and savory salmon dish glazed with a delicate maple coating and cooked to perfection under the broiler.

INGREDIENTS:

- 2 salmon fillets (5 oz / 140 g each)
- 2 tablespoons pure maple syrup (30 mL)
- 1 teaspoon olive oil (5 mL)
- 1/2 teaspoon Dijon mustard (optional, 2.5 mL)
- 1 clove garlic, minced (3 g)
- 1/4 teaspoon ground black pepper (0.5 g)

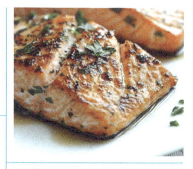

INSTRUCTIONS:

1. Combine the maple syrup, olive oil, black pepper, minced garlic, and Dijon mustard (if using) in a small bowl.
2. Put the salmon fillets in a plastic bag that can be closed or in a shallow plate. Make sure the fillets are uniformly covered after pouring the marinade over them. Let them marinate in the refrigerator for at least 15 minutes.
3. Preheat your oven to high. Place the oven rack approximately 6 inches away from the heat source. Grease and line a baking pan with foil.
4. Put the marinated salmon fillets on the prepared baking sheet, skin-side down. Brush the fillets with any remaining marinade. The salmon should be cooked through and flake readily with a fork after 10 minutes of broiling.
5. Transfer the salmon from the oven and let it rest for 2 minutes before serving. Optionally, garnish with fresh parsley or a lemon wedge.

NUTRITIONAL:
Calories: 250
Protein: 23 g
Fat: 10 g
Carbohydrates: 10 g
Sodium: 40 mg
Potassium: 300 mg
Phosphorus: 200 mg

HERBED TILAPIA FILLET

 **PREP TIME:** 10 minutes    **COOK TIME:** 10 minutes   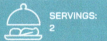 **SERVINGS:** 2

A light and flavorful fish dish with tilapia fillets seasoned with fresh herbs and garlic.

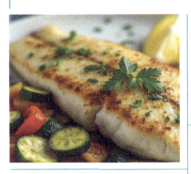

INGREDIENTS:

- 2 tilapia fillets (5 oz / 140 g each)
- 1 tablespoon olive oil (15 mL)
- 1/2 teaspoon garlic powder (1 g)
- 1 tablespoon fresh parsley, chopped (4 g)
- 1/4 teaspoon ground black pepper (0.5 g)

INSTRUCTIONS:

1. Reheat the oven to 375°F or heat a non-stick skillet over medium heat.
2. Apply olive oil to the tilapia fillets on both sides. Sprinkle garlic powder, chopped parsley, and black pepper evenly over the fillets.
3. Put the fillets on a baking pan coated with one sheet of parchment paper and bake them for 10 to 12 minutes or until they become opaque and flake easily with a knife.
4. If pan-searing, place the fillets in the preheated skillet and cook for 4-5 minutes per side or until the fish is fully cooked.
5. Serve warm with a side of vegetables or a light salad.

NUTRITIONAL:
Calories: 160
Protein: 22 g
Fat: 7 g
Carbohydrates: 0 g
Sodium: 40 mg
Potassium: 280 mg
Phosphorus: 200 mg

BAKED COD WITH YOGURT AND MUSHROOMS

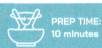 **PREP TIME:** 10 minutes   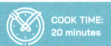 **COOK TIME:** 20 minutes   **SERVINGS:** 2

A creamy and savory baked cod dish with a light yogurt sauce and earthy mushrooms.

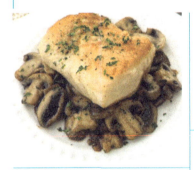

INGREDIENTS:

- 2 cod fillets (5 oz / 140 g each)
- 1/2 cup plain unsweetened yogurt (120 mL)
- 1/2 cup sliced mushrooms (50 g)
- 1 tablespoon olive oil (15 mL)
- 1 clove garlic, minced (3 g)
- 1/4 teaspoon ground black pepper (0.5 g)
- 1 tablespoon fresh parsley, chopped (4 g)

INSTRUCTIONS:

1. Preheat the oven to 375°F. Lightly grease a baking pan with some olive oil.
2. Arrange the cod fillets in the baking pan.
3. In a small bowl, mix the yogurt, minced garlic, black pepper, and half of the chopped parsley.
4. Spread the yogurt mixture evenly over the cod fillets.
5. Scatter the sliced mushrooms around the fillets in the baking dish.
6. Roast the cod for 20 minutes or when the fish becomes opaque and flakes easily with a knife.
7. Remove from the oven and let it rest for 2 minutes.
8. Garnish with the remaining parsley before serving.

NUTRITIONAL:
Calories: 180
Protein: 24 g
Fat: 7 g
Carbohydrates: 4 g
Sodium: 60 mg
Potassium: 290 mg
Phosphorus: 200 mg

GRILLED LEMON GARLIC SHRIMP SKEWERS

 **PREP TIME:** 10 minutes   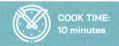 **COOK TIME:** 10 minutes   **SERVINGS:** 2

A light and flavorful shrimp dish marinated with lemon, garlic, and parsley, perfect for grilling.

INGREDIENTS:

- 8 oz shrimp, peeled and deveined (225 g)
- 1 tablespoon olive oil (15 mL)
- 1 clove garlic, minced (3 g)
- 1 tablespoon lemon juice (15 mL)
- 1 tablespoon fresh parsley, chopped (4 g)

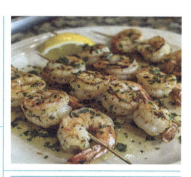

INSTRUCTIONS:

1. To create the marinade, combine the olive oil, lemon juice, chopped parsley, and minced garlic in a small bowl.
2. Pour the marinade over the shrimp in a shallow dish or resealable plastic bag. Ensure the shrimp are evenly coated. Marinate in the refrigerator for 15 minutes.
3. To avoid scorching, immerse wooden skewers in water for ten to fifteen minutes. Thread the marinated shrimp onto the skewers.
4. Reheat a grill or grill pan over medium heat.
5. The shrimp should be pink in color, opaque, and cooked after 2 to 3 minutes on each side of the skewers.
6. Transfer the skewers from the grill and let them rest for 1-2 minutes before serving.

NUTRITIONAL:
Calories: 180
Protein: 22 g
Fat: 7 g
Carbohydrates: 1 g
Sodium: 110 mg
Potassium: 200 mg
Phosphorus: 180 mg

CRUNCHY OVEN-FRIED CATFISH

 **PREP TIME:** 10 minutes   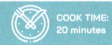 **COOK TIME:** 20 minutes   **SERVINGS:** 2

A healthier take on fried catfish with a crispy coating, baked to golden perfection.

INGREDIENTS:

- 2 catfish fillets (5 oz / 140 g each)
- 1/4 cup breadcrumbs (30 g, kidney-friendly and low-sodium)
- 1 tablespoon olive oil (15 mL)
- 1/2 teaspoon garlic powder (1 g)
- 1/4 teaspoon paprika (0.5 g)
- 1/4 teaspoon ground black pepper (0.5 g)
- 1/2 teaspoon dried parsley (1 g)

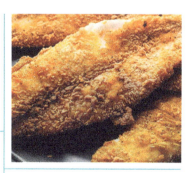

INSTRUCTIONS:

1. Reheat the oven to 400°F and line a baking pan with one sheet of parchment paper or lightly grease it.
2. In a shallow dish, mix breadcrumbs, garlic powder, paprika, black pepper, and dried parsley.
3. Brush each side of the catfish fillets with olive oil. Press each fillet into the breadcrumb mixture to coat it evenly on both sides.
4. Put the coated fillets on the prepared baking sheet.
5. Roast for around 20 minutes, flipping halfway through or until the coating becomes golden and crispy, and the fish flakes easily with a knife.
6. Remove from the oven and let the fillets cool slightly before serving.

NUTRITIONAL:
Calories: 210
Protein: 22 g
Fat: 8 g
Carbohydrates: 7 g
Sodium: 40 mg
Potassium: 200 mg
Phosphorus: 180 mg

BROILED HALIBUT WITH DILL

PREP TIME:
10 minutes

COOK TIME:
10 minutes

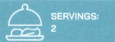
SERVINGS:
2

A delicate and flavorful halibut dish infused with fresh dill and a hint of lemon.

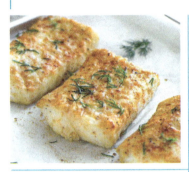

INGREDIENTS:

- 2 halibut fillets (5 oz / 140 g each)
- 1 tablespoon olive oil (15 mL)
- 1 tablespoon fresh dill, chopped (4 g)
- 1 tablespoon lemon juice (15 mL)
- 1/4 teaspoon ground black pepper (0.5 g)

INSTRUCTIONS:

1. Reheat the broiler and position the oven rack about 6 inches from the heat source. Line a baking pan with foil and grease it with some olive oil.
2. Combine the lemon juice, black pepper, chopped dill, and olive oil in a small bowl.
3. Brush the halibut fillets with the dill mixture, ensuring they are evenly coated on both sides.
4. Put the fillets on the prepared baking sheet.
5. Broil for 8-10 minutes or until the halibut is opaque and flakes easily with a knife.
6. Before serving, take the fillets out of the oven and allow them to rest for two minutes.

NUTRITIONAL:
Calories: 200
Protein: 24 g
Fat: 10 g
Carbohydrates: 1 g
Sodium: 50 mg
Potassium: 300 mg
Phosphorus: 220 mg

LOW-SODIUM FISH TACOS

PREP TIME:
10 minutes

COOK TIME:
10 minutes

SERVINGS:
2

A light and flavorful taco featuring tender fish, crunchy cabbage, and a kidney-friendly twist.

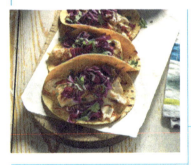

INGREDIENTS:

- 2 white fish fillets (5 oz / 140 g each, such as cod or tilapia)
- 1 tablespoon olive oil (15 mL)
- 1/2 teaspoon garlic powder (1 g)
- 1 cup shredded cabbage (75 g)
- 4 small low-sodium tortillas (6-inch, 50 g each)
- Optional garnish: fresh parsley, lemon wedge

INSTRUCTIONS:

1. Preheat a skillet over medium heat.
2. Brush the fish fillets with olive oil and season both sides evenly with garlic powder and black pepper if desired.
3. After adding the fillets to the pan, cook for three to four minutes on each side or until opaque and easily flaked with a fork. After 2 minutes, take the fish out of the pan and set it aside to rest.
4. Warm the low-sodium tortillas in a separate dry skillet or in the microwave for a few seconds to soften.
5. Assemble the tacos by flaking the cooked fish into chunks and placing it onto the tortillas. Top with shredded cabbage.
6. For extra taste, sprinkle with fresh parsley or squeeze of lemon juice and serve right away.

NUTRITIONAL:
Calories: 240
Protein: 24 g
Fat: 8 g
Carbohydrates: 18 g
Sodium: 60 mg
Potassium: 220 mg
Phosphorus: 190 mg

PINA COLADA SHRIMP WITH BROWN RICE

 **PREP TIME:** 10 minutes

 **COOK TIME:** 10 minutes

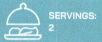 **SERVINGS:** 2

A tropical-inspired dish featuring tender shrimp in a creamy coconut pineapple sauce served over brown rice.

INGREDIENTS:

For the Shrimp:
- 8 oz shrimp, peeled and deveined (225 g)
- 1 tablespoon olive oil (15 mL)
- 60 milliliters (about 1/4 cup) of unsweetened coconut milk
- 60 milliliters, or 1/4 cup, of unsweetened pineapple juice
- 1 clove garlic, minced (3 g)
- 1/4 teaspoon ground black pepper (0.5 g)

For the Rice:
- 1/2 cup uncooked brown rice (85 g)
- 1 cup water or low-sodium broth (240 mL)

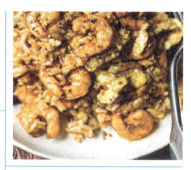

INSTRUCTIONS:

1. Rinse the brown rice under cold water.
2. Boil some water or low-sodium broth in a small saucepan. Simmer the rice for 20-25 minutes, covered, over low heat, or until it is soft and absorbs all of the liquid. Set aside.
3. A big skillet over medium heat should be used to heat the olive oil. Once the shrimp are pink and opaque, add them to the pan and cook for two to three minutes on each side. Put the shrimp aside after taking them out of the pan.
4. Put the minced garlic into the same pan and cook for a minute or until it starts to smell good.
5. Blend in the pineapple juice and coconut milk. Let the sauce thicken slightly by simmering for 3-4 minutes.
6. Toss the shrimp with the sauce again after returning them to the pan. Cook for 1-2 minutes to heat through.
7. Divide the cooked brown rice between two plates.
8. Top the rice with the pina colada shrimp and spoon the sauce over the dish.
9. Garnish with fresh parsley or a small wedge of lime if desired.

Calories: 310
Protein: 20 g
Fat: 8 g
Carbohydrates: 38 g
Sodium: 65 mg
Potassium: 250 mg
Phosphorus: 220 mg

NUTRITIONAL:

EGGPLANT SEAFOOD CASSEROLE

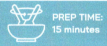 **PREP TIME:** 15 minutes

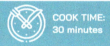 **COOK TIME:** 30 minutes

 SERVINGS: 2

A hearty and flavorful casserole with tender eggplant, a medley of seafood, and a light herb seasoning.

INGREDIENTS:

- 1 medium eggplant, diced (300 g)
- 6 oz shrimp, peeled and deveined (170 g)
- 4 oz white fish, such as cod or tilapia, diced (115 g)
- 1 tablespoon olive oil (15 mL)
- 1 clove garlic, minced (3 g)
- 1/4 teaspoon dried oregano (0.5 g)
- 1/4 teaspoon ground black pepper (0.5 g)
- 60 milliliters (or 1/4 cup) of low-sodium chicken broth
- 1 tablespoon fresh parsley, chopped (4 g)

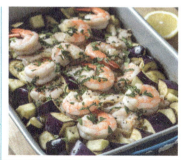

INSTRUCTIONS:

1. Start the oven to 375°F and lightly grease a casserole dish with olive oil.
2. Warm the olive oil in the pan above medium heat. Incorporate the diced eggplant and sauté for 5-7 minutes, stirring intermittently, until tender.
3. Add the minced garlic, dried oregano, and ground black pepper to the skillet. Thoroughly mix and fry for one minute until aromatic.
4. Stir in the low-sodium chicken broth and cook for 2 minutes. Remove from heat.
5. Arrange the cooked eggplant in an even layer in the casserole dish. Top with the diced white fish and shrimp.
6. Envelop the dish with aluminum foil and bake for 20-25 minutes, or until the seafood is thoroughly cooked and the shrimp are pink and opaque.
7. After taking the casserole out of the oven, top it with chopped parsley and set it aside to rest for 5 minutes.

Calories: 200
Protein: 20 g
Fat: 7 g
Carbohydrates: 10 g
Sodium: 120 mg
Potassium: 350 mg
Phosphorus: 220 mg

NUTRITIONAL:

BAKED WHITEFISH WITH VEGETABLES

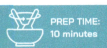 **PREP TIME:** 10 minutes

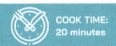 **COOK TIME:** 20 minutes

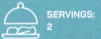 **SERVINGS:** 2

A simple and healthy dish featuring tender whitefish fillets baked with zucchini and carrots, lightly seasoned with thyme and black pepper.

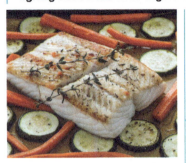

INGREDIENTS:

- 2 whitefish fillets (5 oz / 140 g each, such as cod or tilapia)
- 1 medium zucchini, sliced into rounds (200 g)
- 1 medium carrot, julienned (70 g)
- 1 tablespoon olive oil (15 mL)
- 1/2 teaspoon dried thyme (1 g)
- 1/4 teaspoon ground black pepper (0.5 g)

INSTRUCTIONS:

1. Start the oven to 375°F and lightly grease a baking dish with olive oil.
2. Make a bed for the fish in the baking dish by arranging the sliced zucchini and julienned carrots.
3. Place the whitefish fillets on top of the vegetables.
4. Apply a drizzle of the olive oil over the fish and vegetables. Sprinkle with dried thyme and black pepper.
5. Place foil over the dish and bake for fifteen minutes.
6. Once the fish becomes opaque and flakes readily when tested with a fork, remove the cover and continue baking for another 5 minutes.
7. Two minutes of resting time should be allowed before serving. Plate the fish with the baked vegetables and enjoy.

NUTRITIONAL:
Calories: 200
Protein: 22 g
Fat: 8 g
Carbohydrates: 4 g
Sodium: 45 mg
Potassium: 280 mg
Phosphorus: 200 mg

HALIBUT WITH LEMON CAPER SAUCE

 PREP TIME: 10 minutes

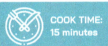 **COOK TIME:** 15 minutes

 SERVINGS: 2

A light and elegant dish with tender halibut topped with a tangy lemon caper sauce.

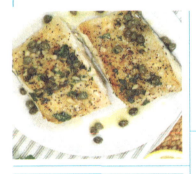

INGREDIENTS:

- 2 halibut fillets (5 oz / 140 g each)
- 1 tablespoon olive oil (15 mL)
- 1 clove garlic, minced (3 g)
- 1 tablespoon lemon juice (15 mL)
- 1 tablespoon capers, rinsed and drained (15 g)
- 1/4 teaspoon ground black pepper (0.5 g)
- 1 tablespoon fresh parsley, chopped (4 g)

INSTRUCTIONS:

1. Preheat a skillet over medium heat. Add half of the olive oil.
2. Season the halibut fillets with black pepper and place them in the skillet. Cook for 4-5 minutes per side or until the fish is opaque and flakes easily with a fork. Take the fillets out of the pan and put them aside.
3. Put the minced garlic and more olive oil into the same pan. Sauté for 1 minute until fragrant.
4. After scraping out any browned remains from the skillet's bottom, stir in the capers and lemon juice. Keep it low for a minute or two to let the flavors meld.
5. After the halibut has been cooked, put it back in the pan and top the fillets with the lemon caper sauce. Heat for an additional minute.
6. When ready to serve, take it off the fire and top with chopped fresh parsley.

NUTRITIONAL:
Calories: 200
Protein: 24 g
Fat: 8 g
Carbohydrates: 1 g
Sodium: 50 mg
Potassium: 280 mg
Phosphorus: 200 mg

MEDITERRANEAN GRILLED SWORDFISH

PREP TIME:
10 minutes

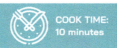
COOK TIME:
10 minutes

SERVINGS:
2

A flavorful and hearty dish with swordfish steaks marinated in a Mediterranean-inspired blend of olive oil, oregano, garlic, and lemon juice.

INGREDIENTS:

- 2 swordfish steaks (6 oz / 170 g each)
- 1 tablespoon olive oil (15 mL)
- 1/2 teaspoon dried oregano (1 g)
- 1 clove garlic, minced (3 g)
- 1 tablespoon lemon juice (15 mL)
- 1/4 teaspoon ground black pepper (0.5 g)

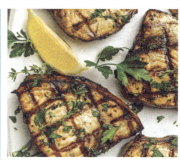

INSTRUCTIONS:

1. Combine the olive oil, dried oregano, minced garlic, some lemon juice, and black pepper in a small bowl and whisk to combine.
2. In the shallow dish or a plastic bag that can be sealed, lay the swordfish steaks. Coat the fish thoroughly on both sides by pouring the marinade over it. For a minimum of fifteen minutes, marinate the fish in the fridge.
3. Put a grill or pan on high heat to get it ready to cook. For nonstick cooking, lightly oil the pan or grill grates.
4. Remove the swordfish steaks from the marinade, allowing any excess to drip off. Discard the remaining marinade.
5. Grill the swordfish steaks for 4-5 minutes per side or until they are firm and opaque and the internal temperature reaches 145°F.
6. After taking it off the grill, give it two minutes to rest.
7. Serve warm, optionally garnished with lemon wedges or fresh parsley.

Calories: 270
Protein: 32 g
Fat: 12 g
Carbohydrates: 1 g
Sodium: 50 mg
Potassium: 300 mg
Phosphorus: 250 mg

NUTRITIONAL:

STEAMED MUSSELS WITH GARLIC

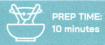
PREP TIME:
10 minutes

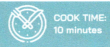
COOK TIME:
10 minutes

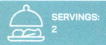
SERVINGS:
2

A light and flavorful dish of tender mussels steamed with garlic, parsley, and a touch of lemon.

INGREDIENTS:

- 1 lb fresh mussels, cleaned and debearded (450 g)
- 1 tablespoon olive oil (15 mL)
- 2 cloves garlic, minced (6 g)
- 2 tablespoons fresh parsley, chopped (8 g)
- 1 tablespoon lemon juice (15 mL)
- (60 mL) of low-sodium vegetable broth or 1/4 cup of water

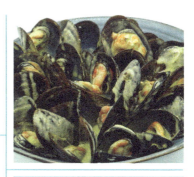

INSTRUCTIONS:

1. Toss the olive oil into a large covered saucepan and set over medium heat. Add the minced garlic and sauté for 1-2 minutes until fragrant.
2. After cleaning, place the mussels in the pot and gently mix them with the garlic and olive oil.
3. Pour in the water or low-sodium vegetable broth and cover the pot with a lid. Increase the heat to medium-high.
4. Steam the mussels for 5-7 minutes or until the shells open. Shake the pot gently once or twice during cooking to ensure even steaming. Discard any mussels that remain closed.
5. Take the saucepan off the stove and mix in the parsley and lemon juice. Just toss the mussels around a little to coat them in the delicious liquid.
6. Serve immediately with the broth ladled over the mussels.

Calories: 200
Protein: 22 g
Fat: 8 g
Carbohydrates: 4 g
Sodium: 60 mg
Potassium: 250 mg
Phosphorus: 200 mg

NUTRITIONAL:

WARM SEAFOOD SALAD

 **PREP TIME:** 15 minutes

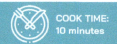 **COOK TIME:** 10 minutes

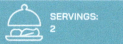 **SERVINGS:** 2

A delightful and light salad with tender seafood and crisp greens served warm with a zesty dressing.

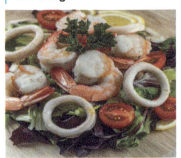

NUTRITIONAL:

Calories: 210
Protein: 24 g
Fat: 8 g
Carbohydrates: 6 g
Sodium: 110 mg
Potassium: 250 mg
Phosphorus: 200 mg

INGREDIENTS:

- 6 oz shrimp, peeled and deveined (170 g)
- 4 oz scallops or squid rings (115 g)
- 1 tablespoon olive oil (15 mL)
- 1 clove garlic, minced (3 g)
- 1/4 teaspoon ground black pepper (0.5 g)
- 2 cups mixed salad greens (100 g)
- 75 grams, or half a cup, of cherry tomatoes
- 1 tablespoon lemon juice (15 mL)
- 1 tablespoon fresh parsley, chopped (4 g)

INSTRUCTIONS:

1. Warm some olive oil in the pan over medium heat. Add the minced garlic and sauté for 1 minute until fragrant.
2. Add the shrimp and scallops (or squid) to the skillet. Cook for 2-3 minutes per side or until the shrimp turn pink and the scallops are opaque. Sprinkle with black pepper. Remove from heat.
3. Toss the salad greens and cherry tomatoes halves in a large basin.
4. Arrange the warm seafood over the greens.
5. A simple dressing may be made by mixing fresh parsley with lemon juice in a small bowl. Drizzle the dressing over the salad.
6. Toss gently to combine and serve immediately.

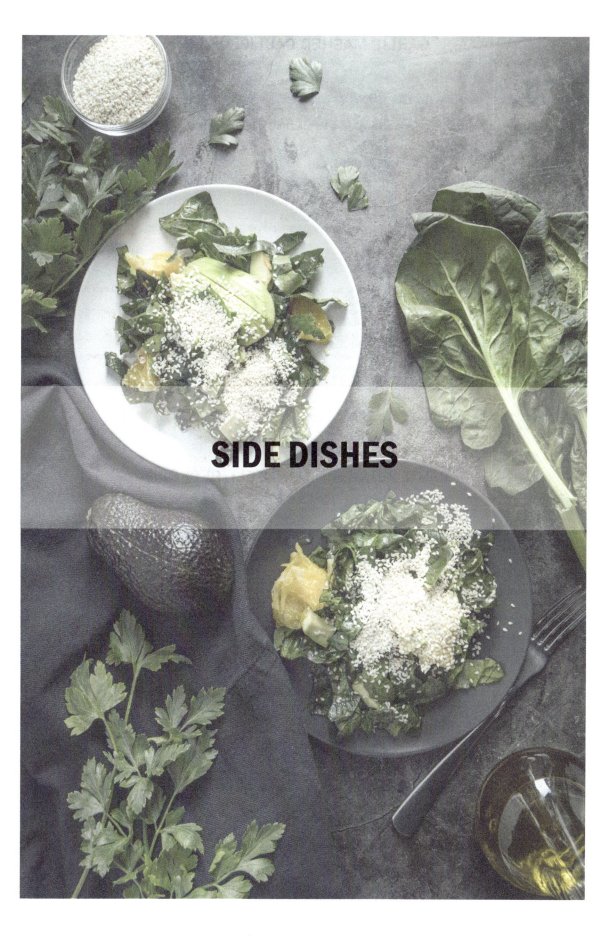

SIDE DISHES

GARLIC MASHED CAULIFLOWER

 **PREP TIME:** 10 minutes 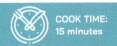 **COOK TIME:** 15 minutes 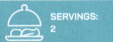 **SERVINGS:** 2

A creamy and flavorful low-carb alternative to mashed potatoes infused with garlic and olive oil.

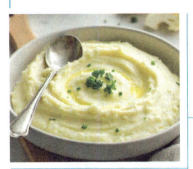

INGREDIENTS:

- 2 cups cauliflower florets (200 g)
- (60 mL) of unsweetened almond milk, 1/4 cup
- 1 tablespoon olive oil (15 mL)
- 1 clove garlic, minced (3 g)
- 1/4 teaspoon ground black pepper (0.5 g)

INSTRUCTIONS:

1. Get some water boiling in a saucepan. Sauté the cauliflower florets for 10 to 12 minutes or until they are really soft. Drain well.
2. Warm some olive oil in a small skillet over medium heat. Add the minced garlic and sauté for 1-2 minutes until fragrant.
3. Blend or process the cooked cauliflower with the garlic and olive oil that has been sautéed. Add the unsweetened almond milk. Blend until smooth.
4. Season with black pepper and blend again to combine. To get the desired consistency, add additional almond milk.
5. Put the mashed cauliflower in a bowl and warm it up before serving.

NUTRITIONAL:
Calories: 80
Protein: 2 g
Fat: 6 g
Carbohydrates: 5 g
Sodium: 30 mg
Potassium: 200 mg
Phosphorus: 60 mg

ROASTED ZUCCHINI AND BELL PEPPERS

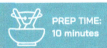 **PREP TIME:** 10 minutes  **COOK TIME:** 10 minutes   **SERVINGS:** 2

A simple and flavorful vegetable side dish featuring tender zucchini and bell peppers roasted with garlic and thyme.

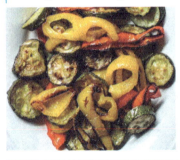

INGREDIENTS:

- 1 medium zucchini, sliced into rounds (200 g)
- 120 grams (1 medium red bell pepper) sliced
- 1 tablespoon olive oil (15 mL)
- 1/2 teaspoon garlic powder (1 g)
- 1/4 teaspoon dried thyme (0.5 g)

INSTRUCTIONS:

1. Start the oven to 400°F and line a baking sheet with parchment paper.
2. Place the zucchini slices and red bell pepper strips in a large mixing bowl.
3. Apply a drizzle of olive oil over the vegetables and sprinkle with garlic powder and dried thyme. Toss to coat evenly.
4. Arrange the veggies on the baking pan in a single layer.
5. To produce soft and slightly browned vegetables, roast them in the oven for 18 to 20 minutes, turning once halfway through.
6. Remove from the oven and let cool for a minute before serving warm.

NUTRITIONAL:
Calories: 90
Protein: 2 g
Fat: 7 g
Carbohydrates: 6 g
Sodium: 20 mg
Potassium: 200 mg
Phosphorus: 30 mg

HERBED RICE PILAF

 **PREP TIME:** 5 minutes   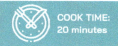 **COOK TIME:** 20 minutes   **SERVINGS:** 2

A light and aromatic rice dish flavored with parsley, garlic, and olive oil.

INGREDIENTS:

- 1/2 cup uncooked white rice (85 g)
- 1 tablespoon olive oil (15 mL)
- 1 clove garlic, minced (3 g)
- 1 tablespoon fresh parsley, chopped (4 g)
- 1/4 teaspoon ground black pepper (0.5 g)
- 1 cup water or low-sodium broth (240 mL)

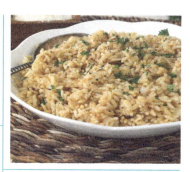

INSTRUCTIONS:

1. Warm some olive oil in a small saucepan over medium heat.
2. Add the minced garlic and sauté for 1 minute until fragrant.
3. Stir in the uncooked white rice and cook for 1-2 minutes, stirring frequently, to lightly toast the grains.
4. Pour in the water or low-sodium broth and bring to a boil.
5. Lower the temperature to a low setting, cover the pot, and let it simmer for fifteen minutes, or until the rice is ready and all of the liquid has been absorbed.
6. Remove the saucepan from the heat and let it sit, covered, for 5 minutes.
7. Warm the rice, fluff it with a fork, then toss in the chopped parsley and black pepper.

Calories: 180
Protein: 3 g
Fat: 7 g
Carbohydrates: 26 g
Sodium: 10 mg
Potassium: 50 mg
Phosphorus: 35 mg

NUTRITIONAL:

STEAMED GREEN BEANS WITH LEMON

 **PREP TIME:** 5 minutes   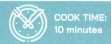 **COOK TIME:** 10 minutes   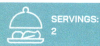 **SERVINGS:** 2

A fresh and simple side dish featuring tender green beans lightly seasoned with lemon and olive oil.

INGREDIENTS:

- 2 cups green beans, trimmed (200 g)
- 1 tablespoon olive oil (15 mL)
- 1 tablespoon lemon juice (15 mL)
- 1/4 teaspoon ground black pepper (0.5 g)

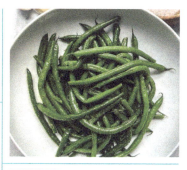

INSTRUCTIONS:

1. Fill a pot with a few inches of water and place a steamer basket inside. Bring the water to a boil.
2. Cover the steamer basket, add the green beans, and steam for five to seven minutes, or until the beans are soft but slightly crunchy.
3. After steaming, take the green beans out of the pot and place them in a serving dish.
4. Then, top the green beans with the olive oil and squeeze some lemon juice. Sprinkle with black pepper and toss gently to coat.
5. Serve warm as a light and refreshing side dish.

Calories: 80
Protein: 2 g
Fat: 7 g
Carbohydrates: 4 g
Sodium: 5 mg
Potassium: 150 mg
Phosphorus: 30 mg

NUTRITIONAL:

CARROT AND PARSNIP MASH

 **PREP TIME:** 10 minutes

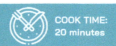 **COOK TIME:** 20 minutes

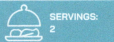 **SERVINGS:** 2

A creamy and slightly sweet mash made with carrots and parsnips, perfect as a healthy side dish.

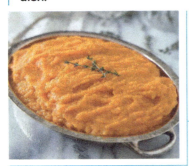

INGREDIENTS:

- 2 medium carrots, peeled and chopped (150 g)
- 2 medium parsnips, peeled and chopped (150 g)
- 1 tablespoon olive oil (15 mL)
- (60 mL) of unsweetened almond milk, 1/4 cup
- 1/4 teaspoon ground black pepper (0.5 g)

INSTRUCTIONS:

1. Get some water boiling in a saucepan. Add the chopped carrots and parsnips and cook for 15-20 minutes, or until both are tender and easily pierced with a fork.
2. Drain the carrots and parsnips and transfer them to a large mixing bowl.
3. Add the olive oil, unsweetened almond milk, and black pepper to the bowl.
4. To make a smooth puree, mash the veggies with a potato masher or try an immersion blender. To have a creamier consistency, simply add additional almond milk.
5. Adjust seasoning with additional black pepper if needed.
6. Serve warm as a flavorful and nutritious side dish.

NUTRITIONAL:

Calories: 120
Protein: 2 g
Fat: 7 g
Carbohydrates: 13 g
Sodium: 15 mg
Potassium: 250 mg
Phosphorus: 40 mg

OVEN-ROASTED SWEET POTATO CUBES (LIMITED)

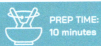 **PREP TIME:** 10 minutes

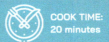 **COOK TIME:** 20 minutes

 SERVINGS: 2

A delicious and slightly sweet roasted sweet potato side dish seasoned with paprika and parsley.

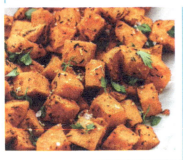

INGREDIENTS:

- 1 small cup of peeled and cubed sweet potato (150 g, portioned out)
- 1 tablespoon olive oil (15 mL)
- 1/2 teaspoon paprika (1 g)
- 1 tablespoon fresh parsley, chopped (4 g)

INSTRUCTIONS:

1. Start the oven to 400°F and line a baking sheet with parchment paper.
2. Whisk together the paprika, sweet potato cubes, and olive oil in a big basin. Toss to coat the sweet potatoes evenly.
3. On the baking sheet that has been preheated, evenly distribute the sweet potatoes that have been seasoned.
4. Roast the sweet potatoes in the oven for 18 to 20 minutes, turning them over halfway through the cooking process until they are soft and have a light caramelization.
5. Immediately after removing it from the oven, garnish the dish with chopped parsley before serving.
6. Serve warm as a flavorful side dish.

NUTRITIONAL:

Calories: 110
Protein: 1 g
Fat: 7 g
Carbohydrates: 10 g
Sodium: 10 mg
Potassium: 150 mg
Phosphorus: 25 mg

CUCUMBER AND DILL SALAD

 **PREP TIME:** 10 minutes

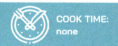 **COOK TIME:** none

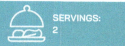 **SERVINGS:** 2

A refreshing and light salad with crisp cucumber and fragrant dill, perfect as a quick side dish.

INGREDIENTS:

- 2 medium cucumbers, peeled and thinly sliced (200 g)
- 1 tablespoon fresh dill, chopped (4 g)
- 1 tablespoon olive oil (15 mL)
- 1 tablespoon lemon juice (15 mL)
- 1/4 teaspoon ground black pepper (0.5 g)

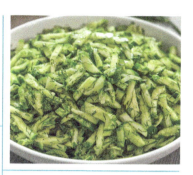

INSTRUCTIONS:

1. Throw the sliced cucumber and peeled cucumber into a big bowl with the chopped dill.
2. Mix the dressing ingredients (olive oil, lemon juice, and black pepper) in a small bowl.
3. Coat the cucumbers equally by pouring the dressing over them and gently tossing them.
4. Give the salad 5 minutes to settle so the flavors can combine.
5. As a light and refreshing side dish, serve chilled or at room temperature.

NUTRITIONAL:
Calories: 80
Protein: 1 g
Fat: 7 g
Carbohydrates: 3 g
Sodium: 5 mg
Potassium: 120 mg
Phosphorus: 20 mg

ZUCCHINI NOODLES WITH GARLIC

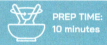 **PREP TIME:** 10 minutes

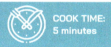 **COOK TIME:** 5 minutes

 SERVINGS: 2

A simple and healthy dish featuring zucchini noodles lightly sautéed with garlic and parsley.

INGREDIENTS:

- 2 medium zucchinis, spiralized (200 g)
- 1 tablespoon olive oil (15 mL)
- 1 clove garlic, minced (3 g)
- 1 tablespoon fresh parsley, chopped (4 g)
- 1/4 teaspoon ground black pepper (0.5 g, optional)

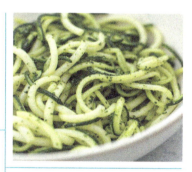

INSTRUCTIONS:

1. Warm some olive oil in the large skillet over medium heat.
2. Toss in the minced garlic and cook for a minute or two or until it starts to release its aroma.
3. Gently stir in the spiralized zucchini with the garlic and olive oil in the skillet.
4. To achieve a texture that is both soft and slightly crunchy, cook the zucchini for two to three minutes, stirring once or twice.
5. Take the skillet off the stove and, if you like, top the zucchini noodles with some chopped parsley and black pepper.
6. Serve warm as a light side dish or a base for other toppings.

NUTRITIONAL:
Calories: 80
Protein: 1 g
Fat: 7 g
Carbohydrates: 3 g
Sodium: 5 mg
Potassium: 150 mg
Phosphorus: 20 mg

CABBAGE STIR-FRY

 **PREP TIME:** 5 minutes   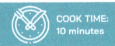 **COOK TIME:** 10 minutes    **SERVINGS:** 2

A quick and simple stir-fry featuring tender cabbage seasoned with garlic and black pepper.

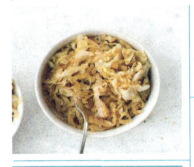

INGREDIENTS:

- 2 cups shredded cabbage (200 g)
- 1 tablespoon olive oil (15 mL)
- 1 clove garlic, minced (3 g)
- 1/4 teaspoon ground black pepper (0.5 g)

INSTRUCTIONS:

1. Warm some olive oil in the large skillet or wok over medium heat.
2. Toss in the minced garlic and cook for a minute or two or until it starts to release its aroma.
3. Toss the shredded cabbage with the olive oil and garlic in the skillet.
4. Stir-fry the cabbage for 5-7 minutes, stirring occasionally, until it is tender but still slightly crisp.
5. Sprinkle with black pepper and stir to combine.
6. For a fast and nutritious side dish, take it off the burner and serve it warm.

NUTRITIONAL:
Calories: 80
Protein: 1 g
Fat: 7 g
Carbohydrates: 3 g
Sodium: 5 mg
Potassium: 120 mg
Phosphorus: 25 mg

CAULIFLOWER FRIED RICE

 **PREP TIME:** 10 minutes    **COOK TIME:** 10 minutes   **SERVINGS:** 2

A light and flavorful low-carb alternative to traditional fried rice, made with riced cauliflower and simple seasonings.

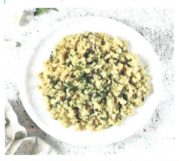

INGREDIENTS:

- 2 cups riced cauliflower (200 g)
- 1 tablespoon olive oil (15 mL)
- 1 clove garlic, minced (3 g)
- 1 tablespoon fresh parsley, chopped (4 g)
- 1/4 teaspoon ground black pepper (0.5 g)

INSTRUCTIONS:

1. Warm some olive oil in the large skillet or wok over medium heat.
2. Toss in the minced garlic and cook for a minute or two or until it starts to release its aroma.
3. Simmer the riced cauliflower for 5 to 7 minutes, tossing it around every so often or until it becomes soft and slightly browned.
4. Stir in the chopped parsley and black pepper, mixing well to combine.
5. Take it off the fire and enjoy it warm as a side or for topping other low-carb dishes.

NUTRITIONAL:
Calories: 90
Protein: 2 g
Fat: 7 g
Carbohydrates: 5 g
Sodium: 5 mg
Potassium: 150 mg
Phosphorus: 30 mg

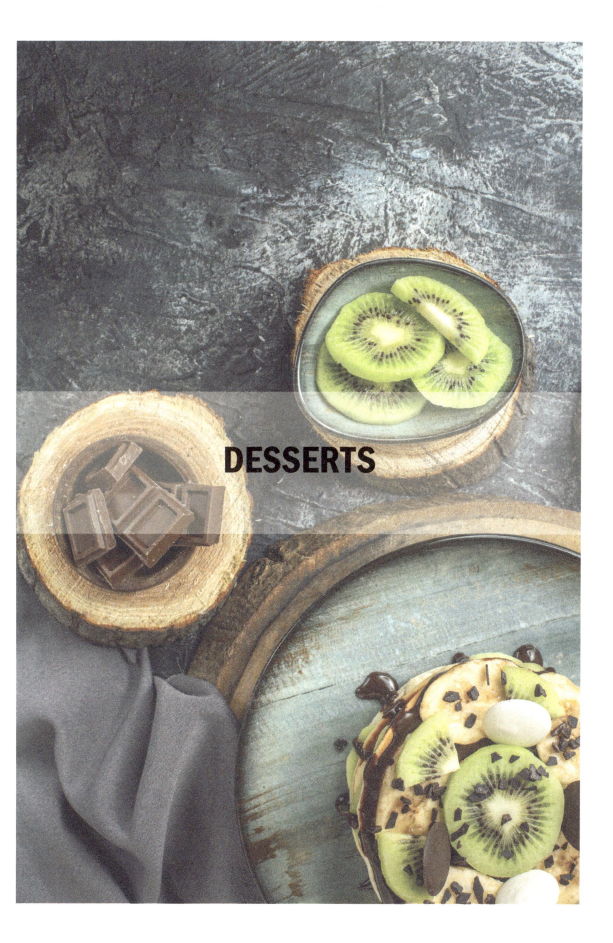

DESSERTS

APPLE CINNAMON COMPOTE

 PREP TIME: 10 minutes 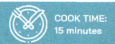 COOK TIME: 15 minutes 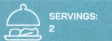 SERVINGS: 2

A warm and comforting compote with tender apples and the delightful aroma of cinnamon.

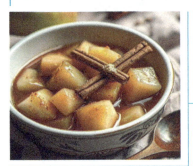

INGREDIENTS:

- 2 medium apples, peeled, cored, and diced (200 g)
- 1/2 teaspoon ground cinnamon (1 g)
- 1/4 cup water (60 mL)
- 1 teaspoon honey or kidney-friendly sweetener (optional, 5 mL)

INSTRUCTIONS:

1. Place the diced apples in a small saucepan.
2. Add the water, ground cinnamon, and honey if using. Stir to combine.
3. After about ten to fifteen minutes of stirring occasionally over medium heat, the apples should be soft, and the sauce should have thickened slightly.
4. After a few minutes, take the compote off the heat.
5. You may eat it warm or cold, and it goes well with yogurt, cereal, or as a side dish.

NUTRITIONAL:
Calories: 80
Protein: 0 g
Fat: 0 g
Carbohydrates: 21 g
Sodium: 2 mg
Potassium: 150 mg
Phosphorus: 10 mg

BLUEBERRY ALMOND MILK POPSICLES

 PREP TIME: 10 minutes   COOK TIME: 4-6 hours   SERVINGS: 4

A refreshing and creamy treat with the natural sweetness of blueberries and a hint of vanilla.

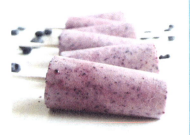

INGREDIENTS:

- 1 cup fresh blueberries (150 g)
- 1 cup unsweetened almond milk (240 mL)
- 1/2 teaspoon vanilla extract (2.5 mL)

INSTRUCTIONS:

1. Place the blueberries, almond milk, and vanilla extract in a blender. Blend until smooth.
2. Pour the mixture evenly into popsicle molds, leaving a little space at the top to allow for expansion.
3. Insert popsicle sticks into the molds.
4. Freeze for 4-6 hours or until fully set.
5. To remove the popsicles from the molds, run them briefly under warm water.
6. Serve immediately and enjoy a healthy, refreshing dessert.

NUTRITIONAL:
Calories: 30
Protein: 1 g
Fat: 1 g
Carbohydrates: 5 g
Sodium: 10 mg
Potassium: 50 mg
Phosphorus: 10 mg

RICE PUDDING WITH VANILLA

 **PREP TIME:** 5 minutes

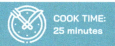 **COOK TIME:** 25 minutes

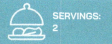 **SERVINGS:** 2

A creamy and comforting dessert with the rich flavor of vanilla, perfect for any occasion.

INGREDIENTS:

- 2 medium zucchini, diced (400 g)
- 2 cloves garlic, minced (6 g)
- 1 tablespoon olive oil (15 mL)
- 4 cups low-sodium vegetable broth (1 L)
- 1 tablespoon fresh parsley, chopped (4 g)
- 1/2 teaspoon fresh thyme leaves (1 g)

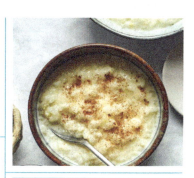

INSTRUCTIONS:

1. The cooked rice and almond milk should be combined in the medium saucepan.
2. Stirring occasionally, cook for 15-20 minutes over medium heat or until mixture reaches a creamy consistency.
3. Stir in the vanilla extract and sugar if using. Cook for an additional 2-3 minutes.
4. Allow the pudding to cool slightly after removing it from the heat.
5. Serve warm or chilled, optionally garnished with a sprinkle of cinnamon or fresh fruit.

Calories: 80
Protein: 1 g
Fat: 2 g
Carbohydrates: 15 g
Sodium: 10 mg
Potassium: 50 mg
Phosphorus: 20 mg

NUTRITIONAL:

STRAWBERRY GELATIN DESSERT

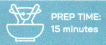 **PREP TIME:** 15 minutes

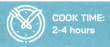 **COOK TIME:** 2-4 hours

 SERVINGS: 4

A delightful treat that is both light and refreshing, created with your choice of natural sweetener and fresh strawberries.

INGREDIENTS:

- 1 cup fresh strawberries, hulled and chopped (150 g)
- 1 packet unflavored gelatin (7 g)
- 1 cup water, divided (240 mL)
- 1 teaspoon sugar or kidney-friendly sweetener (optional, 5 g)

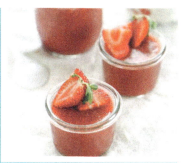

INSTRUCTIONS:

1. Pour a quarter cup of water over the flavorless gelatin in a small bowl and set aside for 5 minutes to bloom.
2. Put the remaining 3/4 cup of water and, if using, sugar into a saucepan. Heat over medium heat until the sugar dissolves and the water is warm but not boiling.
3. Stir the bloomed gelatin into the warm water mixture until completely dissolved.
4. Place the chopped strawberries into a blender and blend until smooth.
5. Pour the strawberry puree into the gelatin mixture and stir well to combine.
6. Divide the mixture among individual serving dishes or cups.
7. Chill in the refrigerator for 2-4 hours or until set.
8. Serve chilled, optionally garnished with fresh strawberry slices or a dollop of whipped topping.

Calories: 25
Protein: 2 g
Fat: 0 g
Carbohydrates: 4 g
Sodium: 5 mg
Potassium: 40 mg
Phosphorus: 5 mg

NUTRITIONAL:

BAKED CINNAMON PEARS

 PREP TIME:
10 minutes

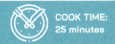 COOK TIME:
25 minutes

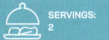 SERVINGS:
2

A warm and comforting dessert with tender baked pears infused with cinnamon and a touch of honey.

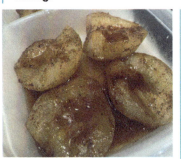

INGREDIENTS:

- 2 medium pears, peeled, halved, and cored (200 g)
- 1/2 teaspoon ground cinnamon (1 g)
- 1 teaspoon honey or kidney-friendly sweetener (5 mL, optional)
- 1/4 cup water (60 mL)

INSTRUCTIONS:

1. Start the oven to 375°F (190°C) and lightly grease a small baking dish.
2. Half the pears, cut the side up, and lay them in the baking dish.
3. Sprinkle the ground cinnamon evenly over the pears. Drizzle the honey on top if using.
4. Pour the water into the bottom of the baking dish to create a steaming effect.
5. Ten minutes in the oven with the foil on top should do the trick.
6. After 5 more minutes of baking, take the foil off to give the tops a little browning.
7. Let the pears cool slightly before serving. Serve warm, optionally garnished with a dollop of yogurt or a sprinkle of chopped nuts.

NUTRITIONAL:
Calories: 90
Protein: 0 g
Fat: 0 g
Carbohydrates: 24 g
Sodium: 2 mg
Potassium: 150 mg
Phosphorus: 10 mg

BERRY CHIA PUDDING

 PREP TIME:
10 minutes

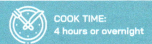 COOK TIME:
4 hours or overnight

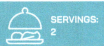 SERVINGS:
2

A creamy and nutritious dessert featuring chia seeds, almond milk, and fresh raspberries, lightly flavored with vanilla.

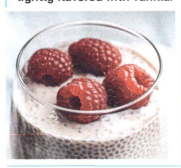

INGREDIENTS:

- 1 cup unsweetened almond milk (240 mL)
- 2 tablespoons chia seeds (30 g, limited)
- 1/2 teaspoon vanilla extract (2.5 mL)
- 1/2 cup fresh raspberries (75 g)

INSTRUCTIONS:

1. All the ingredients—almond milk, chia seeds, and vanilla extract—must be thoroughly mixed in a medium bowl.
2. Cover the bowl and refrigerate for at least 4 hours or overnight, stirring occasionally in the first hour to prevent clumping.
3. Before serving, gently mash half of the fresh raspberries and stir them into the pudding for added flavor.
4. Divide the chia pudding into two serving bowls or glasses.
5. Top each serving with the remaining fresh raspberries. Serve chilled.

NUTRITIONAL:
Calories: 110
Protein: 3 g
Fat: 5 g
Carbohydrates: 10 g
Sodium: 20 mg
Potassium: 80 mg
Phosphorus: 40 mg

BANANA OAT COOKIES

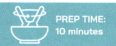 **PREP TIME:** 10 minutes

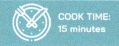 **COOK TIME:** 15 minutes

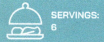 **SERVINGS:** 6

A simple and kidney-friendly treat made with oats, a touch of banana, and a hint of cinnamon.

INGREDIENTS:

- 1/2 cup rolled oats (40 g)
- 2 tablespoons mashed banana (30 g, limited)
- 1/4 teaspoon ground cinnamon (0.5 g)

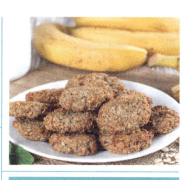

INSTRUCTIONS:

1. Start the oven to 350°F (175°C) and spread parchment paper on a baking pan.
2. In a small bowl, mix the rolled oats, mashed banana, and ground cinnamon until well combined.
3. Form the dough into small balls using a tablespoon scoop and set them on a baking sheet that has been preheated. Press down slightly to flatten them.
4. Bake for 12-15 minutes or until the cookies are firm and lightly golden.
5. After 5 minutes, take the baking sheet out of the oven and set the cookies on a wire rack to cool.
6. Serve as a light snack or dessert.

Calories: 30
Protein: 1 g
Fat: 0.5 g
Carbohydrates: 6 g
Sodium: 1 mg
Potassium: 30 mg
Phosphorus: 10 mg

NUTRITIONAL:

PEACH SORBET

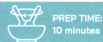 **PREP TIME:** 10 minutes

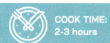 **COOK TIME:** 2-3 hours

 SERVINGS: 4

A light and refreshing sorbet made with fresh peaches, perfect for a kidney-friendly dessert.

INGREDIENTS:

- 2 cups fresh peaches, peeled and diced (300 g)
- 1 tablespoon lemon juice (15 mL)
- 2 tablespoons sugar or kidney-friendly sweetener (optional, 25 g)
- 1/4 cup water (60 mL)

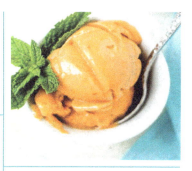

INSTRUCTIONS:

1. Blend or process diced peaches, lemon juice, water, and sugar.
2. Fill a shallow dish or freezer-safe container with the peach mixture.
3. Place the container in the freezer for 2-3 hours, stirring every 30 minutes to prevent large ice crystals from forming.
4. Once the sorbet is firm but scoopable, serve in small bowls or glasses.
5. If you choose, you can add a mint leaf or a slice of fresh peach as a garnish.

Calories: 40
Protein: 0 g
Fat: 0 g
Carbohydrates: 10 g
Sodium: 1 mg
Potassium: 90 mg
Phosphorus: 10 mg

NUTRITIONAL:

VANILLA COCONUT MACAROONS

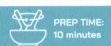 **PREP TIME:** 10 minutes   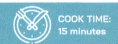 **COOK TIME:** 15 minutes   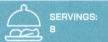 **SERVINGS:** 8

A light and chewy treat made with coconut flakes, egg whites, and a touch of vanilla.

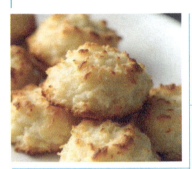

INGREDIENTS:

- 1 cup unsweetened coconut flakes (80 g)
- 2 egg whites (70 g)
- 1/2 teaspoon vanilla extract (2.5 mL)
- 1 teaspoon sugar or kidney-friendly sweetener (optional, 5 g)

INSTRUCTIONS:

1. Start the oven to 325°F (165°C) and spread parchment paper on a baking pan.
2. Whip the egg whites into a foam in a mixing bowl.
3. Gently fold in the coconut flakes, vanilla extract, and sugar, if using, until the mixture is well combined.
4. Make little mounds out of the mixture by spooning it onto the baking sheet that has been lined with parchment paper.
5. Bake for 12-15 minutes or until the edges are golden brown.
6. Transfer the macaroons to a wire rack after cooling for 5 minutes on the baking sheet.
7. Serve as a light and satisfying dessert or snack.

NUTRITIONAL:
Calories: 40
Protein: 1 g
Fat: 3 g
Carbohydrates: 2 g
Sodium: 5 mg
Potassium: 20 mg
Phosphorus: 10 mg

CRANBERRY-APPLE CRISP

 PREP TIME: 15 minutes   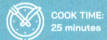 **COOK TIME:** 25 minutes   **SERVINGS:** 2

A warm and comforting dessert with tart cranberries, sweet apples, and a crunchy oat topping.

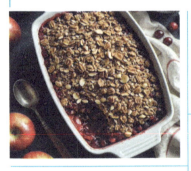

INGREDIENTS:

- 1 medium apple, peeled, cored, and sliced (150 g)
- 1/2 cup fresh cranberries (50 g)
- 1/4 cup rolled oats (20 g)
- 1/2 teaspoon ground cinnamon (1 g)
- 1 tablespoon honey or kidney-friendly sweetener (15 mL)

INSTRUCTIONS:

1. Start the oven to 350°F (175°C) and spread parchment paper on a baking pan.
2. Put the fresh cranberries and cut apples in a bowl and stir to incorporate. Drizzle with half the honey and sprinkle with half the cinnamon. Toss to coat evenly, then spread the mixture in the baking dish.
3. In the same bowl, mix the rolled oats, remaining cinnamon, and the rest of the honey until combined.
4. Divide the oat mixture among the baking dish's fruit slices and sprinkle them evenly.
5. After 20 to 25 minutes in the oven, the fruit should be soft and the topping should be golden.
6. Before serving warm, allow the crisp to cool for a few minutes.

NUTRITIONAL:
Calories: 110
Protein: 2 g
Fat: 1 g
Carbohydrates: 24 g
Sodium: 5 mg
Potassium: 70 mg
Phosphorus: 30 mg

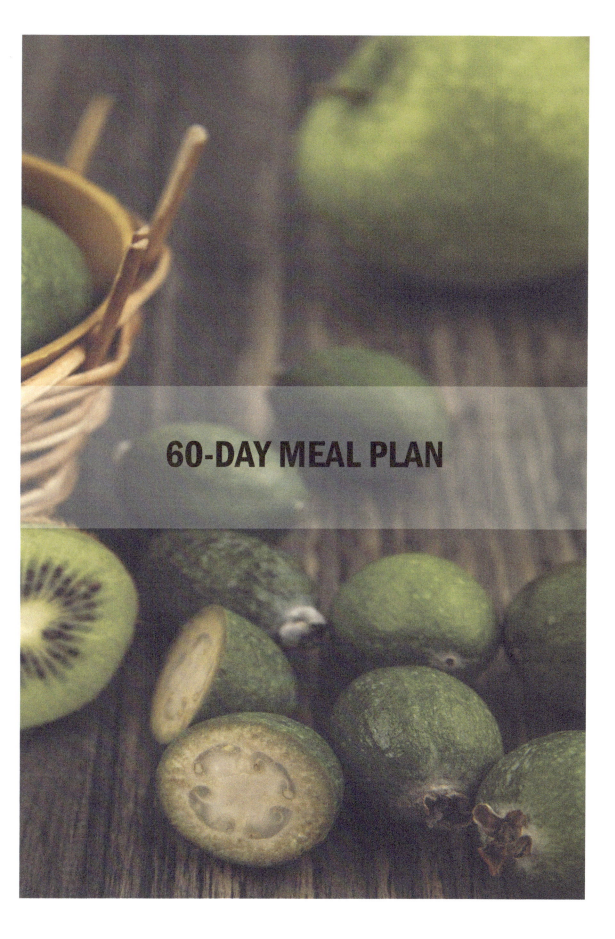

60-DAY MEAL PLAN

60-DAY MEAL PLAN

Each daily meal plan serves as a FOUNDATION of the diet but does not include specific side dishes for lunch and dinner. The choice of side dishes is left to the reader and their doctor, although suggested options are provided in a separate column.

Each recipe includes calorie content and key nutrients essential for individuals with kidney disease. Readers should determine their allowable intake with their doctor, based on their weight and health condition, and then calculate the appropriate portion sizes.

Day	Breakfast	Lunch	Dinner	Dessert	Side Dish/Salad
1	Blueberry Oatmeal	Grilled Lemon Herb Chicken	Baked Cod with Yogurt and Mushrooms	Baked Cinnamon Pears	Steamed Green Beans with Lemon
2	Egg White Scramble with Herbs	Turkey and Green Bean Stir-Fry	Lemon Pepper Pork Chops	Berry Chia Pudding	Cucumber and Dill Salad
3	Cinnamon French Toast	Zucchini and Herb Soup	Beef Bourguignon	Apple Cinnamon Compote	Roasted Zucchini and Bell Peppers
4	Smoothie Bowl	Herbed Tilapia Fillet	Mediterranean Grilled Swordfish	Peach Sorbet	Cauliflower Fried Rice
5	Vanilla Rice Pudding	Stuffed Bell Peppers with Beef	Steamed Mussels with Garlic	Cranberry-Apple Crisp	Herbed Rice Pilaf
6	Sweet Potato Hash	Baked Whitefish with Vegetables	Herbed Lamb Patties	Vanilla Coconut Macaroons	Warm Seafood Salad
7	Fruit Salad	Chicken and Rice Soup	Turkey and Carrot Stew	Rice Pudding with Vanilla	Carrot and Parsnip Mash
8	Chia Berry Pudding	Roasted Zucchini and Bell Peppers	Slow-Cooked Pulled Pork	Banana Oat Cookies	Steamed Broccoli with Garlic
9	Cucumber Avocado Wrap	Beef and Zucchini Skillet	Barley and Vegetable Soup	Strawberry Gelatin Dessert	Oven-Roasted Sweet Potato Cubes (Limited)
10	Breakfast Muffins	Herb-Crusted Chicken Tenders	Cabbage Stir-Fry with Grilled Chicken	Blueberry Almond Milk Popsicles	Zucchini Noodles with Garlic
11	Blueberry Oatmeal	Grilled Lemon Herb Chicken	Baked Cod with Yogurt and Mushrooms	Baked Cinnamon Pears	Steamed Green Beans with Lemon
12	Egg White Scramble with Herbs	Turkey and Green Bean Stir-Fry	Lemon Pepper Pork Chops	Berry Chia Pudding	Cucumber and Dill Salad
13	Cinnamon French Toast	Zucchini and Herb Soup	Beef Bourguignon	Apple Cinnamon Compote	Roasted Zucchini and Bell Peppers
14	Smoothie Bowl	Herbed Tilapia Fillet	Mediterranean Grilled Swordfish	Peach Sorbet	Cauliflower Fried Rice
15	Vanilla Rice Pudding	Stuffed Bell Peppers with Beef	Steamed Mussels with Garlic	Cranberry-Apple Crisp	Herbed Rice Pilaf
16	Sweet Potato Hash	Baked Whitefish with Vegetables	Herbed Lamb Patties	Vanilla Coconut Macaroons	Warm Seafood Salad
17	Fruit Salad	Chicken and Rice Soup	Turkey and Carrot Stew	Rice Pudding with Vanilla	Carrot and Parsnip Mash
18	Chia Berry Pudding	Roasted Zucchini and Bell Peppers	Slow-Cooked Pulled Pork	Banana Oat Cookies	Steamed Broccoli with Garlic

19	Cucumber Avocado Wrap	Beef and Zucchini Skillet	Barley and Vegetable Soup	Strawberry Gelatin Dessert	Oven-Roasted Sweet Potato Cubes (Limited)
20	Breakfast Muffins	Herb-Crusted Chicken Tenders	Cabbage Stir-Fry with Grilled Chicken	Blueberry Almond Milk Popsicles	Zucchini Noodles with Garlic
21	Blueberry Oatmeal	Grilled Lemon Herb Chicken	Baked Cod with Yogurt and Mushrooms	Baked Cinnamon Pears	Steamed Green Beans with Lemon
22	Egg White Scramble with Herbs	Turkey and Green Bean Stir-Fry	Lemon Pepper Pork Chops	Berry Chia Pudding	Cucumber and Dill Salad
23	Cinnamon French Toast	Zucchini and Herb Soup	Beef Bourguignon	Apple Cinnamon Compote	Roasted Zucchini and Bell Peppers
24	Smoothie Bowl	Herbed Tilapia Fillet	Mediterranean Grilled Swordfish	Peach Sorbet	Cauliflower Fried Rice
25	Vanilla Rice Pudding	Stuffed Bell Peppers with Beef	Steamed Mussels with Garlic	Cranberry-Apple Crisp	Herbed Rice Pilaf
26	Sweet Potato Hash	Baked Whitefish with Vegetables	Herbed Lamb Patties	Vanilla Coconut Macaroons	Warm Seafood Salad
27	Fruit Salad	Chicken and Rice Soup	Turkey and Carrot Stew	Rice Pudding with Vanilla	Carrot and Parsnip Mash
28	Chia Berry Pudding	Roasted Zucchini and Bell Peppers	Slow-Cooked Pulled Pork	Banana Oat Cookies	Steamed Broccoli with Garlic
29	Cucumber Avocado Wrap	Beef and Zucchini Skillet	Barley and Vegetable Soup	Strawberry Gelatin Dessert	Oven-Roasted Sweet Potato Cubes (Limited)
30	Breakfast Muffins	Herb-Crusted Chicken Tenders	Cabbage Stir-Fry with Grilled Chicken	Blueberry Almond Milk Popsicles	Zucchini Noodles with Garlic
31	Blueberry Oatmeal	Grilled Lemon Herb Chicken	Baked Cod with Yogurt and Mushrooms	Baked Cinnamon Pears	Steamed Green Beans with Lemon
32	Egg White Scramble with Herbs	Turkey and Green Bean Stir-Fry	Lemon Pepper Pork Chops	Berry Chia Pudding	Cucumber and Dill Salad
33	Cinnamon French Toast	Zucchini and Herb Soup	Beef Bourguignon	Apple Cinnamon Compote	Roasted Zucchini and Bell Peppers
34	Smoothie Bowl	Herbed Tilapia Fillet	Mediterranean Grilled Swordfish	Peach Sorbet	Cauliflower Fried Rice
35	Vanilla Rice Pudding	Stuffed Bell Peppers with Beef	Steamed Mussels with Garlic	Cranberry-Apple Crisp	Herbed Rice Pilaf
36	Sweet Potato Hash	Baked Whitefish with Vegetables	Herbed Lamb Patties	Vanilla Coconut Macaroons	Warm Seafood Salad
37	Fruit Salad	Chicken and Rice Soup	Turkey and Carrot Stew	Rice Pudding with Vanilla	Carrot and Parsnip Mash
38	Chia Berry Pudding	Roasted Zucchini and Bell Peppers	Slow-Cooked Pulled Pork	Banana Oat Cookies	Steamed Broccoli with Garlic
39	Cucumber Avocado Wrap	Beef and Zucchini Skillet	Barley and Vegetable Soup	Strawberry Gelatin Dessert	Oven-Roasted Sweet Potato Cubes (Limited)

40	Breakfast Muffins	Herb-Crusted Chicken Tenders	Cabbage Stir-Fry with Grilled Chicken	Blueberry Almond Milk Popsicles	Zucchini Noodles with Garlic
41	Blueberry Oatmeal	Grilled Lemon Herb Chicken	Baked Cod with Yogurt and Mushrooms	Baked Cinnamon Pears	Steamed Green Beans with Lemon
42	Egg White Scramble with Herbs	Turkey and Green Bean Stir-Fry	Lemon Pepper Pork Chops	Berry Chia Pudding	Cucumber and Dill Salad
43	Cinnamon French Toast	Zucchini and Herb Soup	Beef Bourguignon	Apple Cinnamon Compote	Roasted Zucchini and Bell Peppers
44	Smoothie Bowl	Herbed Tilapia Fillet	Mediterranean Grilled Swordfish	Peach Sorbet	Cauliflower Fried Rice
45	Vanilla Rice Pudding	Stuffed Bell Peppers with Beef	Steamed Mussels with Garlic	Cranberry-Apple Crisp	Herbed Rice Pilaf
46	Sweet Potato Hash	Baked Whitefish with Vegetables	Herbed Lamb Patties	Vanilla Coconut Macaroons	Warm Seafood Salad
47	Fruit Salad	Chicken and Rice Soup	Turkey and Carrot Stew	Rice Pudding with Vanilla	Carrot and Parsnip Mash
48	Chia Berry Pudding	Roasted Zucchini and Bell Peppers	Slow-Cooked Pulled Pork	Banana Oat Cookies	Steamed Broccoli with Garlic
49	Cucumber Avocado Wrap	Beef and Zucchini Skillet	Barley and Vegetable Soup	Strawberry Gelatin Dessert	Oven-Roasted Sweet Potato Cubes (Limited)
50	Breakfast Muffins	Herb-Crusted Chicken Tenders	Cabbage Stir-Fry with Grilled Chicken	Blueberry Almond Milk Popsicles	Zucchini Noodles with Garlic
51	Blueberry Oatmeal	Grilled Lemon Herb Chicken	Baked Cod with Yogurt and Mushrooms	Baked Cinnamon Pears	Steamed Green Beans with Lemon
52	Egg White Scramble with Herbs	Turkey and Green Bean Stir-Fry	Lemon Pepper Pork Chops	Berry Chia Pudding	Cucumber and Dill Salad
53	Cinnamon French Toast	Zucchini and Herb Soup	Beef Bourguignon	Apple Cinnamon Compote	Roasted Zucchini and Bell Peppers
54	Smoothie Bowl	Herbed Tilapia Fillet	Mediterranean Grilled Swordfish	Peach Sorbet	Cauliflower Fried Rice
55	Vanilla Rice Pudding	Stuffed Bell Peppers with Beef	Steamed Mussels with Garlic	Cranberry-Apple Crisp	Herbed Rice Pilaf
56	Sweet Potato Hash	Baked Whitefish with Vegetables	Herbed Lamb Patties	Vanilla Coconut Macaroons	Warm Seafood Salad
57	Fruit Salad	Chicken and Rice Soup	Turkey and Carrot Stew	Rice Pudding with Vanilla	Carrot and Parsnip Mash
58	Chia Berry Pudding	Roasted Zucchini and Bell Peppers	Slow-Cooked Pulled Pork	Banana Oat Cookies	Steamed Broccoli with Garlic
59	Cucumber Avocado Wrap	Beef and Zucchini Skillet	Barley and Vegetable Soup	Strawberry Gelatin Dessert	Oven-Roasted Sweet Potato Cubes (Limited)
60	Breakfast Muffins	Herb-Crusted Chicken Tenders	Cabbage Stir-Fry with Grilled Chicken	Blueberry Almond Milk Popsicles	Zucchini Noodles with Garlic

WEEK 1

Vegetables

- Carrot: 1 medium (70 g)
- Zucchini: 1 medium (200 g)
- Green beans: 1 cup (100 g)
- Celery: 3 stalks (150 g)
- Onion: 2 medium (200 g)
- Garlic: 7 cloves (21 g)
- Red bell pepper: 1/2 cup (80 g)
- Cucumber: 1 large (200 g)
- Fresh parsley: 10 tablespoons (40 g)
- Fresh thyme: 2 teaspoons (4 g)
- Baby spinach: 1 cup (30 g)
- Cherry tomatoes: 1/2 cup (75 g)
- Radishes: 1/2 cup (50 g)
- Cabbage: 3 cups (225 g)

Fruits

- Blueberries: 3/4 cup (120 g)
- Strawberries: 1 cup (160 g)
- Apple: 3 medium (450 g)
- Pineapple: 1/4 cup (50 g)
- Banana: 1 medium (120 g)

Grains & Legumes

- Quinoa: 1/2 cup uncooked (85 g)
- White rice: 3/4 cup uncooked (127.5 g)
- Rolled oats: 1 cup (80 g)
- All-purpose flour: 1 1/4 cups (150 g)
- Low-sodium tortilla: 2 pieces (60 g)
- Low-sodium bread: 4 slices (120 g)

Proteins

- Egg whites: 16 large (480 mL)
- Chicken breast (boneless, skinless): 3 pieces (420 g)
- Turkey breast: 8 oz (225 g)
- Tofu: 1/2 block (150 g)

Dairy Alternatives

- Unsweetened almond milk: 5 1/4 cups (1.26 L)
- Coconut milk: 1/4 cup (60 mL)

Oils, Spices, and Condiments

- Olive oil: 8 tablespoons (120 mL)
- Lemon juice: 4 teaspoons (20 mL)
- Dijon mustard: 1 tablespoon (15 mL)
- Honey: 1 tablespoon (15 mL)
- Ground cinnamon: 3/4 teaspoon (1.5 g)
- Garlic powder: 1/4 teaspoon (0.3 g)
- Black pepper: 1 teaspoon (2 g)
- Baking powder: 1 teaspoon (4 g)
- Curry powder: 1 teaspoon (2 g)
- Balsamic vinegar: 2 teaspoons (10 mL)
- Apple cider vinegar: 2 teaspoons (10 mL)
- Vanilla extract: 1/4 teaspoon (1.25 mL)

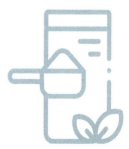

WEEK 2

Vegetables

- Zucchini: 4 medium (800 g)
- Bell peppers: 2 (200 g)
- Broccoli: 1 bunch (200 g)
- Carrot: 1 medium (70 g)
- Green beans: 1 cup (100 g)
- Sweet potato: 2 medium (400 g)
- Cabbage: 2 cups (200 g)
- Garlic: 6 cloves (18 g)
- Onion: 2 medium (200 g)
- Fresh dill: 1 tablespoon (4 g)
- Green onion: 2 tablespoons (10 g)
- Fresh parsley: 4 tablespoons (16 g)
- Fresh thyme: 1 tablespoon (4 g)

Fruits

- Blueberries: 1 cup (150 g)
- Strawberries: 1 cup (160 g)
- Banana: 3 medium (360 g)
- Apple: 2 medium (300 g)
- Peaches (for sorbet): 2 (300 g)
- Lemon: 2 (120 g)

Grains & Legumes

- Rolled oats: 1/2 cup (40 g)
- Quinoa: 1/2 cup uncooked (85 g)
- Barley: 1/4 cup uncooked (50 g)
- All-purpose flour: 1/4 cup (30 g)
- Low-sodium bread: 1 slice (30 g)

Proteins

- Egg whites: 8 large (240 mL)
- Chicken breast (boneless, skinless): 3 pieces (420 g)
- Pork (for slow-cooking): 1 lb (450 g)
- Ground beef: 1/2 lb (225 g)
- Tilapia fillets: 2 (250 g)
- Herb-crusted chicken tenders: 4 (200 g)

Dairy Alternatives

- Unsweetened almond milk: 2 cups (480 mL)

Oils, Spices, and Condiments

- Olive oil: 8 tablespoons (120 mL)
- Ground cinnamon: 1 teaspoon (2 g)
- Black pepper: 1 teaspoon (2 g)
- Garlic powder: 1/2 teaspoon (1 g)
- Ground ginger: 1/4 teaspoon (1 g)
- Cumin: 1/4 teaspoon (1 g)
- Balsamic vinegar: 1 tablespoon (15 mL)
- Dijon mustard: 1 tablespoon (15 mL)
- Honey: 1 tablespoon (15 mL)
- Vinegar (apple cider): 1 teaspoon (5 mL)

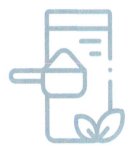

WEEK 3

Vegetables

- Zucchini: 4 medium (800 g)
- Bell peppers: 4 (400 g)
- Sweet potatoes: 4 medium (800 g)
- Broccoli: 1 bunch (200 g)
- Carrots: 4 medium (280 g)
- Parsnips: 2 medium (300 g)
- Green beans: 1 cup (100 g)
- Cabbage: 2 cups (200 g)
- Garlic: 6 cloves (18 g)
- Onion: 3 medium (300 g)
- Fresh parsley: 5 tablespoons (20 g)
- Fresh thyme: 2 tablespoons (8 g)
- Fresh dill: 2 teaspoons (8 g)
- Green onion: 2 tablespoons (10 g)

Fruits

- Blueberries: 2 cups (300 g)
- Strawberries: 2 cups (320 g)
- Banana: 4 medium (480 g)
- Apples (for crisp and rice pudding): 2 medium (300 g)
- Lemon: 2 (120 g)
- Cranberries (for crisp): 1/2 cup (75 g)

Grains & Legumes

- Rolled oats: 1/2 cup (40 g)
- Quinoa: 1/2 cup uncooked (85 g)
- Rice (for pudding and pilaf): 2 cups (370 g)
- All-purpose flour: 1/2 cup (60 g)
- Barley: 1/4 cup uncooked (50 g)

Proteins

- Egg whites: 8 large (240 mL)
- Chicken breast (boneless, skinless): 4 pieces (560 g)
- Beef (for stuffed peppers): 1 lb (450 g)
- Mussels: 1 lb (450 g)
- Lamb (for patties): 1 lb (450 g)
- Tilapia fillets: 2 (250 g)
- Herb-crusted chicken tenders: 4 (200 g)
- Ground beef (for slow-cooked pork): 1 lb (450 g)

Dairy Alternatives

- Unsweetened almond milk: 2 cups (480 mL)
- Coconut milk: 1/4 cup (60 mL)

Oils, Spices, and Condiments

- Olive oil: 10 tablespoons (150 mL)
- Ground cinnamon: 1 teaspoon (2 g)
- Black pepper: 2 teaspoons (4 g)
- Garlic powder: 1/2 teaspoon (1 g)
- Ground ginger: 1/4 teaspoon (1 g)
- Cumin: 1/4 teaspoon (1 g)
- Balsamic vinegar: 2 tablespoons (30 mL)
- Dijon mustard: 1 tablespoon (15 mL)
- Honey: 1 tablespoon (15 mL)
- Vanilla extract: 1 teaspoon (5 mL)

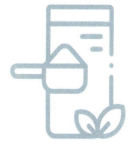

WEEK 4

Vegetables

- Zucchini: 4 medium (800 g)
- Bell peppers: 4 (400 g)
- Sweet potatoes: 4 medium (800 g)
- Broccoli: 1 bunch (200 g)
- Carrots: 4 medium (280 g)
- Parsnips: 2 medium (300 g)
- Green beans: 1 cup (100 g)
- Cabbage: 2 cups (200 g)
- Garlic: 8 cloves (24 g)
- Onion: 4 medium (400 g)
- Fresh parsley: 5 tablespoons (20 g)
- Fresh thyme: 2 tablespoons (8 g)
- Fresh dill: 2 teaspoons (8 g)
- Green onion: 2 tablespoons (10 g)
- Fresh basil: 2 tablespoons (8 g)

Fruits

- Blueberries: 2 cups (300 g)
- Strawberries: 2 cups (320 g)
- Banana: 5 medium (600 g)
- Apples: 2 medium (300 g)
- Peaches (for sorbet): 2 (300 g)
- Cranberries (for crisp): 1/2 cup (75 g)
- Lemon: 2 (120 g)

Grains & Legumes

- Rolled oats: 1/2 cup (40 g)
- Quinoa: 1/2 cup uncooked (85 g)
- Rice (for pudding and pilaf): 3 cups (555 g)
- All-purpose flour: 1/2 cup (60 g)
- Barley: 1/4 cup uncooked (50 g)

Proteins

- Egg whites: 8 large (240 mL)
- Chicken breast (boneless, skinless): 4 pieces (560 g)
- Beef (for stuffed peppers): 1 lb (450 g)
- Mussels: 1 lb (450 g)
- Lamb (for patties): 1 lb (450 g)
- Tilapia fillets: 2 (250 g)
- Herb-crusted chicken tenders: 4 (200 g)
- Ground beef (for slow-cooked pork): 1 lb (450 g)

Dairy Alternatives

- Unsweetened almond milk: 2 cups (480 mL)
- Coconut milk: 1/4 cup (60 mL)

Oils, Spices, and Condiments

- Olive oil: 10 tablespoons (150 mL)
- Ground cinnamon: 1 teaspoon (2 g)
- Black pepper: 2 teaspoons (4 g)
- Garlic powder: 1/2 teaspoon (1 g)
- Ground ginger: 1/4 teaspoon (1 g)
- Cumin: 1/4 teaspoon (1 g)
- Balsamic vinegar: 2 tablespoons (30 mL)
- Dijon mustard: 1 tablespoon (15 mL)
- Honey: 1 tablespoon (15 mL)
- Vanilla extract: 1 teaspoon (5 mL)

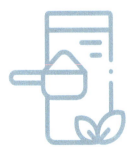

WEEK 5

Vegetables

- Zucchini: 6 medium (1.2 kg)
- Bell peppers: 4 (400 g)
- Sweet potatoes: 4 medium (800 g)
- Broccoli: 1 bunch (200 g)
- Carrots: 4 medium (280 g)
- Parsnips: 2 medium (300 g)
- Green beans: 1 cup (100 g)
- Cabbage: 2 cups (200 g)
- Garlic: 8 cloves (24 g)
- Onion: 4 medium (400 g)
- Fresh parsley: 5 tablespoons (20 g)
- Fresh thyme: 2 tablespoons (8 g)
- Fresh dill: 2 teaspoons (8 g)
- Green onion: 2 tablespoons (10 g)

Fruits

- Blueberries: 2 cups (300 g)
- Strawberries: 2 cups (320 g)
- Banana: 5 medium (600 g)
- Apples: 2 medium (300 g)
- Peaches (for sorbet): 2 (300 g)
- Cranberries (for crisp): 1/2 cup (75 g)
- Lemon: 2 (120 g)

Grains & Legumes

- Rolled oats: 1/2 cup (40 g)
- Quinoa: 1/2 cup uncooked (85 g)
- Rice (for pudding and pilaf): 3 cups (555 g)
- All-purpose flour: 1/2 cup (60 g)
- Barley: 1/4 cup uncooked (50 g)

Proteins

- Egg whites: 8 large (240 mL)
- Chicken breast (boneless, skinless): 4 pieces (560 g)
- Beef (for stuffed peppers): 1 lb (450 g)
- Mussels: 1 lb (450 g)
- Lamb (for patties): 1 lb (450 g)
- Tilapia fillets: 2 (250 g)
- Herb-crusted chicken tenders: 4 (200 g)
- Ground beef (for slow-cooked pork): 1 lb (450 g)

Dairy Alternatives

- Unsweetened almond milk: 2 cups (480 mL)
- Coconut milk: 1/4 cup (60 mL)

Oils, Spices, and Condiments

- Olive oil: 10 tablespoons (150 mL)
- Ground cinnamon: 1 teaspoon (2 g)
- Black pepper: 2 teaspoons (4 g)
- Garlic powder: 1/2 teaspoon (1 g)
- Ground ginger: 1/4 teaspoon (1 g)
- Cumin: 1/4 teaspoon (1 g)
- Balsamic vinegar: 2 tablespoons (30 mL)
- Dijon mustard: 1 tablespoon (15 mL)
- Honey: 1 tablespoon (15 mL)
- Vanilla extract: 1 teaspoon (5 mL)

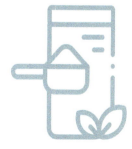

WEEK 6

Vegetables

- Zucchini: 6 medium (1.2 kg)
- Bell peppers: 4 (400 g)
- Sweet potatoes: 4 medium (800 g)
- Broccoli: 1 bunch (200 g)
- Carrots: 4 medium (280 g)
- Parsnips: 2 medium (300 g)
- Green beans: 1 cup (100 g)
- Cabbage: 2 cups (200 g)
- Garlic: 8 cloves (24 g)
- Onion: 4 medium (400 g)
- Fresh parsley: 5 tablespoons (20 g)
- Fresh thyme: 2 tablespoons (8 g)
- Fresh dill: 2 teaspoons (8 g)
- Green onion: 2 tablespoons (10 g)

Fruits

- Blueberries: 2 cups (300 g)
- Strawberries: 2 cups (320 g)
- Banana: 5 medium (600 g)
- Apples: 2 medium (300 g)
- Peaches (for sorbet): 2 (300 g)
- Cranberries (for crisp): 1/2 cup (75 g)
- Lemon: 3 (180 g)

Grains & Legumes

- Rolled oats: 1/2 cup (40 g)
- Quinoa: 1/2 cup uncooked (85 g)
- Rice (for pudding and pilaf): 3 cups (555 g)
- All-purpose flour: 1/2 cup (60 g)
- Barley: 1/4 cup uncooked (50 g)

Proteins

- Egg whites: 8 large (240 mL)
- Chicken breast (boneless, skinless): 4 pieces (560 g)
- Beef (for stuffed peppers): 1 lb (450 g)
- Mussels: 1 lb (450 g)
- Lamb (for patties): 1 lb (450 g)
- Tilapia fillets: 2 (250 g)
- Herb-crusted chicken tenders: 4 (200 g)
- Ground beef (for slow-cooked pork): 1 lb (450 g)

Dairy Alternatives

- Unsweetened almond milk: 2 cups (480 mL)
- Coconut milk: 1/4 cup (60 mL)

Oils, Spices, and Condiments

- Olive oil: 10 tablespoons (150 mL)
- Ground cinnamon: 1 teaspoon (2 g)
- Black pepper: 2 teaspoons (4 g)
- Garlic powder: 1/2 teaspoon (1 g)
- Ground ginger: 1/4 teaspoon (1 g)
- Cumin: 1/4 teaspoon (1 g)
- Balsamic vinegar: 2 tablespoons (30 mL)
- Dijon mustard: 1 tablespoon (15 mL)
- Honey: 1 tablespoon (15 mL)
- Vanilla extract: 1 teaspoon (5 mL)

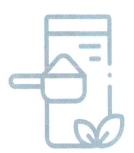

WEEK 7

Vegetables

- Zucchini: 6 medium (1.2 kg)
- Bell peppers: 5 (500 g)
- Sweet potatoes: 4 medium (800 g)
- Broccoli: 1 bunch (200 g)
- Carrots: 4 medium (280 g)
- Parsnips: 2 medium (300 g)
- Green beans: 1 cup (100 g)
- Cabbage: 2 cups (200 g)
- Garlic: 8 cloves (24 g)
- Onion: 4 medium (400 g)
- Fresh parsley: 5 tablespoons (20 g)
- Fresh thyme: 2 tablespoons (8 g)
- Fresh dill: 2 teaspoons (8 g)
- Green onion: 2 tablespoons (10 g)

Fruits

- Blueberries: 2 cups (300 g)
- Strawberries: 2 cups (320 g)
- Banana: 5 medium (600 g)
- Apples: 3 medium (450 g)
- Peaches (for sorbet): 2 (300 g)
- Cranberries (for crisp): 1/2 cup (75 g)
- Lemon: 3 (180 g)

Grains & Legumes

- Rolled oats: 1/2 cup (40 g)
- Quinoa: 1/2 cup uncooked (85 g)
- Rice (for pudding and pilaf): 3 cups (555 g)
- All-purpose flour: 1/2 cup (60 g)
- Barley: 1/4 cup uncooked (50 g)

Proteins

- Egg whites: 8 large (240 mL)
- Chicken breast (boneless, skinless): 4 pieces (560 g)
- Beef (for stuffed peppers): 1 lb (450 g)
- Mussels: 1 lb (450 g)
- Lamb (for patties): 1 lb (450 g)
- Tilapia fillets: 2 (250 g)
- Herb-crusted chicken tenders: 4 (200 g)
- Ground beef (for slow-cooked pork): 1 lb (450 g)

Dairy Alternatives

- Unsweetened almond milk: 2 cups (480 mL)
- Coconut milk: 1/4 cup (60 mL)

Oils, Spices, and Condiments

- Olive oil: 10 tablespoons (150 mL)
- Ground cinnamon: 1 teaspoon (2 g)
- Black pepper: 2 teaspoons (4 g)
- Garlic powder: 1/2 teaspoon (1 g)
- Ground ginger: 1/4 teaspoon (1 g)
- Cumin: 1/4 teaspoon (1 g)
- Balsamic vinegar: 2 tablespoons (30 mL)
- Dijon mustard: 1 tablespoon (15 mL)
- Honey: 1 tablespoon (15 mL)
- Vanilla extract: 1 teaspoon (5 mL)

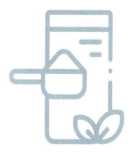

WEEK 8

Vegetables

- Zucchini: 7 medium (1.4 kg)
- Bell peppers: 5 (500 g)
- Sweet potatoes: 4 medium (800 g)
- Broccoli: 1 bunch (200 g)
- Carrots: 4 medium (280 g)
- Parsnips: 2 medium (300 g)
- Green beans: 1 cup (100 g)
- Cabbage: 2 cups (200 g)
- Garlic: 8 cloves (24 g)
- Onion: 4 medium (400 g)
- Fresh parsley: 5 tablespoons (20 g)
- Fresh thyme: 2 tablespoons (8 g)
- Fresh dill: 2 teaspoons (8 g)
- Green onion: 2 tablespoons (10 g)

Fruits

- Blueberries: 2 cups (300 g)
- Strawberries: 2 cups (320 g)
- Banana: 5 medium (600 g)
- Apples: 3 medium (450 g)
- Peaches (for sorbet): 2 (300 g)
- Cranberries (for crisp): 1/2 cup (75 g)
- Lemon: 3 (180 g)

Grains & Legumes

- Rolled oats: 1/2 cup (40 g)
- Quinoa: 1/2 cup uncooked (85 g)
- Rice (for pudding and pilaf): 3 cups (555 g)
- All-purpose flour: 1/2 cup (60 g)
- Barley: 1/4 cup uncooked (50 g)

Proteins

- Egg whites: 8 large (240 mL)
- Chicken breast (boneless, skinless): 4 pieces (560 g)
- Beef (for stuffed peppers): 1 lb (450 g)
- Mussels: 1 lb (450 g)
- Lamb (for patties): 1 lb (450 g)
- Tilapia fillets: 2 (250 g)
- Herb-crusted chicken tenders: 4 (200 g)
- Ground beef (for slow-cooked pork): 1 lb (450 g)

Dairy Alternatives

- Unsweetened almond milk: 2 cups (480 mL)
- Coconut milk: 1/4 cup (60 mL)

Oils, Spices, and Condiments

- Olive oil: 10 tablespoons (150 mL)
- Ground cinnamon: 1 teaspoon (2 g)
- Black pepper: 2 teaspoons (4 g)
- Garlic powder: 1/2 teaspoon (1 g)
- Ground ginger: 1/4 teaspoon (1 g)
- Cumin: 1/4 teaspoon (1 g)
- Balsamic vinegar: 2 tablespoons (30 mL)
- Dijon mustard: 1 tablespoon (15 mL)
- Honey: 1 tablespoon (15 mL)
- Vanilla extract: 1 teaspoon (5 mL)

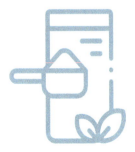

WEEK 9

Vegetables

- Zucchini: 7 medium (1.4 kg)
- Bell peppers: 4 (400 g)
- Sweet potatoes: 4 medium (800 g)
- Broccoli: 1 bunch (200 g)
- Carrots: 5 medium (350 g)
- Parsnips: 2 medium (300 g)
- Green beans: 1 cup (100 g)
- Cabbage: 2 cups (200 g)
- Garlic: 8 cloves (24 g)
- Onion: 4 medium (400 g)
- Fresh parsley: 5 tablespoons (20 g)
- Fresh thyme: 2 tablespoons (8 g)
- Fresh dill: 2 teaspoons (8 g)
- Green onion: 2 tablespoons (10 g)

Fruits

- Blueberries: 2 cups (300 g)
- Strawberries: 2 cups (320 g)
- Banana: 5 medium (600 g)
- Apples: 3 medium (450 g)
- Peaches (for sorbet): 2 (300 g)
- Cranberries (for crisp): 1/2 cup (75 g)
- Lemon: 3 (180 g)

Grains & Legumes

- Rolled oats: 1/2 cup (40 g)
- Quinoa: 1/2 cup uncooked (85 g)
- Rice (for pudding and pilaf): 3 cups (555 g)
- All-purpose flour: 1/2 cup (60 g)
- Barley: 1/4 cup uncooked (50 g)

Proteins

- Egg whites: 8 large (240 mL)
- Chicken breast (boneless, skinless): 4 pieces (560 g)
- Beef (for stuffed peppers): 1 lb (450 g)
- Mussels: 1 lb (450 g)
- Lamb (for patties): 1 lb (450 g)
- Tilapia fillets: 2 (250 g)
- Herb-crusted chicken tenders: 4 (200 g)
- Ground beef (for slow-cooked pork): 1 lb (450 g)

Dairy Alternatives

- Unsweetened almond milk: 2 cups (480 mL)
- Coconut milk: 1/4 cup (60 mL)

Oils, Spices, and Condiments

- Olive oil: 10 tablespoons (150 mL)
- Ground cinnamon: 1 teaspoon (2 g)
- Black pepper: 2 teaspoons (4 g)
- Garlic powder: 1/2 teaspoon (1 g)
- Ground ginger: 1/4 teaspoon (1 g)
- Cumin: 1/4 teaspoon (1 g)
- Balsamic vinegar: 2 tablespoons (30 mL)
- Dijon mustard: 1 tablespoon (15 mL)
- Honey: 1 tablespoon (15 mL)
- Vanilla extract: 1 teaspoon (5 mL)

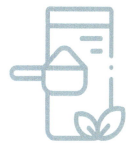

TABLE OF FOOD SUBSTITUTES

Creating a table of food substitutes with sodium, potassium, phosphorus, and protein content per 100 grams of product is an essential step in developing dietary recommendations for elderly individuals with kidney disease. Below is such a table based on available data.

Table of Food Substitutes with Sodium, Potassium, Phosphorus, and Protein Content per 100g:

Original Product	Alternative Product	Sodium (mg)	Potassium (mg)	Phosphorus (mg)	Protein (g)
Salt	Herbs and spices (e.g., basil, oregano)	4-6	50-60	30-40	3-5
	Lemon juice	1	103	16	0.3
	Apple cider vinegar	1	73	8	0
	Nutritional yeast	5	400	300	50
Milk	Rice milk	35	27	15	0.1
	Almond milk	60	50	20	0.5
Cheese	Tofu	7	121	97	8
	Homemade cottage cheese (in moderation)	372	104	190	11.1
Potatoes	Cauliflower	30	299	44	1.9
	Parsnip	10	375	71	1.2
	Pumpkin	1	340	44	1
	Zucchini	3	261	38	1.2
Bananas	Apples	1	107	11	0.3
	Pears	1	116	12	0.4
	Grapes	2	191	20	0.6
	Pineapple	1	109	8	0.5
	Blueberries	1	77	12	0.7
	Strawberries	1	153	24	0.8
Tomatoes	Bell pepper	2	211	26	0.9
	Carrots	69	320	44	0.9
	Beets	78	325	40	1.6
Avocado	Cucumbers	2	147	24	0.7
	Green lettuce	28	194	29	1.4

Eggs	Egg whites	166	163	15	10.9
	Small portions of chicken or fish	70-90	300-400	200-250	20-25
Red meat	Lean chicken or turkey	70-90	300-400	200-250	20-25
	Low-fat fish	60-80	250-350	200-220	18-22
Fatty meat	Lean chicken or turkey	70-90	300-400	200-250	20-25
	Low-fat fish	60-80	250-350	200-220	18-22
Butter	Olive oil	2	1	0	0
	Flaxseed oil	2	0	0	0
Mayonnaise	Homemade yogurt and mustard sauce	200	150	100	3
Fried food	Baked or steamed food	Depends on ingredients	Depends on ingredients	Depends on ingredients	Depends on ingredients
Sugar	Natural sweeteners (stevia, honey)	0	0	0	0
Chocolate	Homemade cocoa and almond milk desserts	50	150	100	2
Wheat flour	Oat flour	2	350	100	13
	Rice flour	0	70	98	5.9

Notes:

- **Sodium:** It is recommended to limit sodium intake, as excess sodium can increase blood pressure and put additional strain on the kidneys.
- **Potassium:** High potassium levels can be dangerous for those with kidney failure, so it is crucial to monitor intake.
- **Phosphorus:** Excess phosphorus consumption can lead to bone and vascular problems in kidney disease patients.
- **Protein:** While protein is essential for the body, excessive amounts can overload the kidneys, so maintaining balance is important.

Data in this table are averaged and may vary depending on the source.

INDEX

Thank you

Thank you so much for purchasing my book! Out of all the options available, you chose this one, and I'm incredibly grateful for that. I appreciate you sticking with it all the way to the end.

Before you go, I have one small request: Would you consider posting a review on the platform? Leaving a review is one of the best and easiest ways to support independent authors like me.

Your feedback not only helps me continue writing books that deliver the results you're looking for, but it also means a great deal to me personally. I'd love to hear your thoughts!